Mini Nutritional Assessment (MNA): Research and Practice in the Elderly

The 1st Nestlé Clinical & Performance Nutrition Workshop, Mini Nutritional Assessment (MNA) – MNA in the Elderly: Research and Practice, *was held in Lausanne, October 1997.*

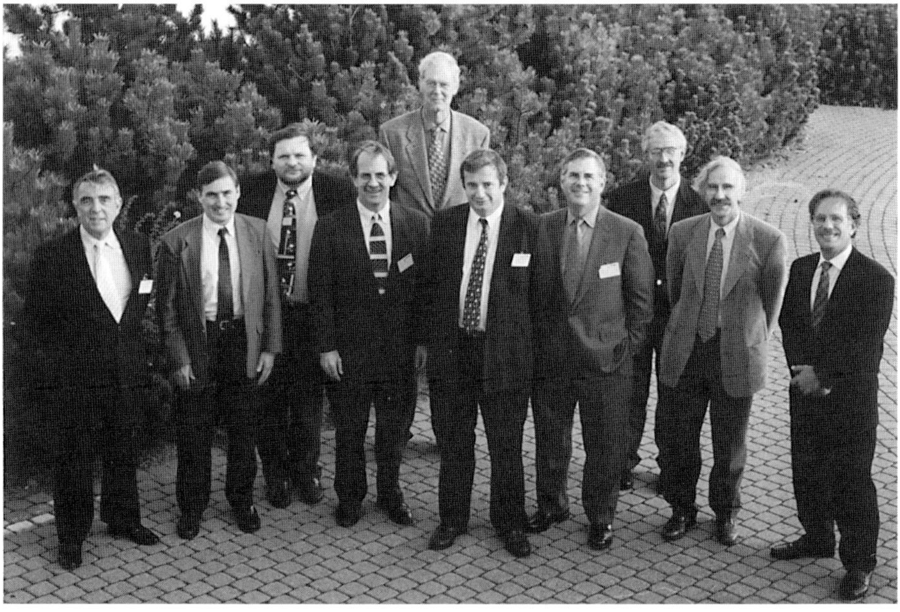

Workshop participants *(left to right):* P. Guesry, A. Salvá, J.E. Morley, D.K. Miller, P. Oster, B. Vellas, Wm.C. Chumlea, E. Schiffrin, Y. Guigoz, L.Z. Rubenstein

Nestlé Nutrition Workshop Series
Clinical & Performance Programme
Volume 1

Mini Nutritional Assessment (MNA): Research and Practice in the Elderly

Editors
Bruno Vellas, University of Toulouse, Toulouse, France
Philip J. Garry, University of New Mexico, Albuquerque, USA
Yves Guigoz, Nestlé Research Center, Lausanne, Switzerland

NESTLÉ NUTRITION SERVICES

Nestlé

KARGER

Nestec Ltd., 55 Avenue Nestlé, CH–1800 Vevey (Switzerland)
S. Karger AG, P.O. Box, CH–4009 Basel (Switzerland)

Printed in Switzerland on acid-free paper by Reinhardt Druck, Basel
ISBN 3–8055–6803–7

Library of Congress Cataloging-in-Publication Data
Mini nutritional assessment (MNA): research and practice in the elderly / editors, Bruno Vellas, Philip J. Garry, Yves Guigoz.
(Nestlé Nutrition workshop series. Clinical & performance programme; v.1)
"Nestlé Nutrition Services."
Includes bibliographical references and index.
ISBN 3–8055–6803–7
1. Nutrition disorders in old age – Diagnosis. 2. Aged – Nutrition – Evaluation. 3. Aged – Diseases – Nutritional aspects. I. Vellas, B.J. (Bruno J.) II. Garry, Philip J., 1933–. III. Guigoz, Yves. IV. Nestlé Nutrition Services. V. Nestlé Clinical & Performance Nutrition Workshop (1st:1997: Lausanne, Switzerland) VI. Series.
RC620.6.M56 1999 618.97′63 – dc21

The material contained in this volume was submitted as previously unpublished material, except in the instances in which credit has been given to the source from which some of the illustrative material was derived.

Great care has been taken to maintain the accuracy of the information contained in the volume. However, neither Nestec Ltd. nor S. Karger AG can be held responsible for errors or for any consequences arising from the use of the information contained herein.

Contents

Preface

The Mini Nutritional Assessment (MNA)[1] as Part of the Geriatric Assessment

The prevalence of malnutrition is high in elderly people in hospital, living in nursing homes, or involved in home care programs. Development of malnutrition in the elderly is usually a continuum, starting with inadequate food intakes, followed by changes in body composition and biochemical variables. Consequences of malnutrition often go unrecognized owing to lack of specific validated instruments to assess nutritional status in frail elderly persons. The Mini Nutritional Assessment (MNA) has recently been designed and validated [1–4] to provide a single, rapid assessment of nutritional status in the elderly. The MNA provides primary care physicians with a tool for rapid screening of patients who may subsequently need a more extensive nutritional assessment. For validation of the MNA we chose to evaluate the tool against the results of nutritional assessment performed by two physicians trained in nutrition, using comprehensive nutritional evaluation (including dietary intakes, anthropometry, and biochemical indices) [1–5]. The MNA was found to be highly correlated with each of these nutritional variables. The sum of the MNA score distinguishes elderly patients with adequate nutritional status (MNA >23.5), protein-energy malnutrition (MNA <17), and at risk of malnutrition (MNA between 17 and 23.5). With this scoring, sensitivity was found to be 96%, specificity 98%, and predictive value 97% [6]. The interobserver MNA score agreement was defined by Cohen's kappa, with a κ value = 0.51 (95% confidence interval 0.28–0.74) [7]. The MNA has been translated into several languages and is used in many clinics around the world. This book reports recent studies on nutrition in the elderly using the MNA and presented at the international meeting on the MNA in the Nestlé Research Center in Lausanne.

B. Vellas, P.J. Garry, Y. Guigoz

[1] The Mini Nutrition Assessment (MNA) form is given in the Appendix.

References

1. Guigoz Y, Vellas BJ, Garry PJ. Assessing the nutritional status of the elderly: the Mini Nutritional Assessment as part of the geriatric evaluation. *Nutr Rev* 1996; 54: S59.
2. Vellas B, Guigoz Y. The Mini Nutritional Assessment. *Facts, research and intervention in geriatrics,* 4th ed. Paris: Springer & Serdi Publishing Co, 1997.
3. Vellas B, Guigoz Y. Nutritional assessment as part of the geriatric evaluation. In: Rubenstein LZ, Bernabei R, Wieland D, eds. *Geriatric assessment technology: state of the arts.* Milan: Kutiz Publishing Co, 1995: 179.
4. Guigoz Y, Vellas B. Malnutrition im Alter: Das Mini Nutritional Assessment (MNA). *Ther Umschau* 1997; 54: 345.
5. Salva A, Bolivar I, Munoz M, Sacristan V. Un nuevo instrumento para la valoración nutricional en geriatría: el Mini Nutritional Assessment (MNA). *Rev Gerontol* 1996; 6: 319.
6. Guigoz Y, Vellas B. Test d'évaluation du statut nutritionnel de la personne âgée: le Mini Nutritional Assessment (MNA). *Med Hyg* 1995; 53: 1965.
7. Gazzoti C, Pepinster A, Petermans J, Albert A. Interobserver agreement on MNA nutritional scale of hospitalized elderly patients. *J Nutr Health Aging* 1997; 1: 23.

Foreword

It has been known for many decades that even in the most affluent countries elderly people admitted to hospital for acute medical or surgical diseases or accidents usually undergo progressive impairment in their nutritional status [1, 2], which remains unnoticed for variable periods. When the medical staff diagnose protein-energy malnutrition, it is often late and may be difficult to correct.

Until 1994, only specialized units in the most advanced geriatric centers were using sophisticated measurements to assess malnutrition and to follow progress during realimentation [3, 4]. The criteria used in different centers were not always the same, making comparison between centers difficult. Moreover the techniques used were specialized and not applicable on a large scale in most geriatric centers, which do not have research personnel among their staff.

Since the beginning of the 1990s, Vellas, Garry, Guigoz and Albarède have developed and validated the Mini Nutritional Assessment (MNA) [5], which is easy, quick, and economical to perform and enables staff to check the nutritional status of elderly people when they enter hospitals or institutions, and to monitor changes occurring during their stay. This allows the necessary nutritional measures to be applied sooner, to prevent a further decline in nutritional status or to restore it to normality.

MNA also allows one to compare the prevalence of protein-energy malnutrition in various centers, and more importantly to compare nutritional measures and protocols used in these centers.

Nestlé Clinical Nutrition is very proud to have supported the development and evaluation of MNA for many years and to have been instrumental in promoting this new and indispensable tool for the better care of the elderly. The MNA Symposium will mark an important step in broadening the use of the MNA tool in its various applications.

Pierre Guesry
Vice-President of Research
Nestlé Research Center,
Lausanne, Switzerland

Franck Arnaud-Battandier
Medical Director
Nestlé Clinical Nutrition,
Sèvres, France

References

1. Mowe M, Bohmer T. The prevalence of undiagnosed protein-calorie undernutrition in a population of 157 hospitalized elderly patients. *J Am Geriatr Soc* 1991; 39: 1089–92.
2. Constans T, Bacq Y, Brechot J-F, Guilmot J-L, Choutet P, Lamisse F. Protein-energy malnutrition in elderly medical patients. *J Am Geriatr Soc* 1992; 40: 263–8.
3. Starker PM. Nutritional assessment of the hospitalized patient. *Adv Nutr Res* 1990; 8: 109–18.
4. Jeejeebhoy KN, Detsky AS, Baker JP. Assessment of nutritional status. *J Parenter Enter Nutr* 1990; 14: 193–6S.
5. Vellas BJ, Guigoz Y, Garry PJ, Albarède JL. The Mini Nutritional Assessment: MNA. In: *Nutrition in the elderly. Facts and research in gerontology 1994* (Supplement). Paris: Serdi, 1994.

Contributors

Speakers

Franck Arnaud-Battandier
Nestlé Clinical Nutrition France
2, Rue Troyon
F–92316 Sèvres Cedex, France

Wm.C. Chumlea
Fels Professor
Wrigth State University
Department of Community Health
and Pediatrics, School of Medicine
1005 Xenia Avenue
Yellow Springs, OH 45387-1695, USA

Robert Cohendy
Département d'Anesthésie-Réanimation
Hôpital Gaston-Doumengue
F–3000 Nîmes Cedex, France

Philip J. Garry
Department of Pathology
School of Medicine
University of New Mexico
2701 Frontier Place
N.E. Room 236
Albuquerque, NM 87131, USA

Martijn Griep
Academic Hospital
Vrije Universiteit Brussel (VUB)
Department of Geriatrics
Laarbeeklaan 101
B–1090 Brussels, Belgium

Pierre Guesry
Nestlé Research Center
Vers-chez-les-Blanc
PO Box 44
CH–1000 Lausanne 26, Switzerland

Yves Guigoz
Nestlé Research Center
Vers-chez-les-Blanc
PO Box 44
CH–1000 Lausanne 26, Switzerland

Douglas K. Miller
School of Medicine
Department of Internal Medicine
Division of Geriatric Medicine
St. Louis University –
Health Sciences Center
1402 S. Grand Blvd., Rm M238
St. Louis, MO 63104, USA

John E. Morley
School of Medicine
Department of Internal Medicine
Division of Geriatric Medicine
St. Louis University –
Health Sciences Center
1402 S. Grand Blvd., Rm M238
St. Louis, MO 63104, USA

Peter Oster
Bethanien Krankenhaus
Geriatrisches Zentrum GmbH
Rohrbachstrasse 149
D–69024 Heidelberg, Germany

Pierluigi Quadri
Ospedale Regionale della Beata Vergine
Via Turconi 23
CH–6850 Mendrisio, Switzerland

Laurence Z. Rubenstein
Director, Geriatric Research Education and Clinical Center (GRECC)
UCLA School of Medicine
VAMC Sepulveda (11E)
16111 Plummer Street
Sepulveda, CA 91343, USA

Antonio Salva I Casanovas
PASS Centre Geriatric Cabanelles
UFISS de Geriatria i Unitat de Convalescencia
RDA Alfonso X, 49-73
E–08304 Mataro (Barcelona), Spain

Kristel Scheirlinckx
Service de gériatrie
Clinique Universitaire de Mont-Godinne
B–5530 Yvoir, Belgium

Eduardo Schiffrin
Nestlé Research Center
Vers-chez-les-Blanc
PO Box 44
CH–1000 Lausanne 26, Switzerland

Bruno Vellas
Service de Médecine Interne et Gérontologique Clinique
Hôpitaux de Toulouse
170, Av. de Casselardit
F–31300 Toulouse, France

Gilbert Zulian
C E S C O
Centre de Soins continus
Chemin de la Savonnière 11
CH–1245 Collonge-Bellerive, Switzerland

Invited Attendees

Giorgetta Cappa / *Italy*
Tommy Cederholm / *Sweden*
Jadwiga Charzewska / *Poland*
Lisette De Groot / *Holland*
Dolf De Ridder / *Belgium*
Hedi Decrey / *Switzerland*
Laura Del Corso / *Italy*
Lorenzo D. Donini / *Italy*
Tamas Fülop Jr. / *Canada*
C. Gazzotti / *Belgium*
R. Gonthier / *France*
Robledo L. Gutierrez / *Mexico*
E. Joosten / *Belgium*
Vladimir Kh. Khavinson / *Russia*
Stefan Krajcik / *Slovakia*
Roman Lutynski / *Poland*
Yoram Maaravi / *Israel*
Irena M. Rea / *N. Ireland*
Michel Roulet / *Switzerland*
Taisa Semesko / *Ukraine*
Lumila Sineok / *Ukraine*
Slavica Suzic / *Yugoslavia*
Orien L. Tulp / *USA*
Raivo Vokk / *Estonia*
Paul Wiesel / *Switzerland*
Ulla Wissing / *Sweden*

Introduction

The New Nestlé Clinical & Performance Nutrition Workshop Series

In 1997, Nestlé created the Nutrition Strategic Business Division (NSBD) in order to centralise and enhance its specific competence in nutrition. Thus, five departments compose this division. Infant and Child Nutrition covers normal and disease-related nutrition for this age group. Clinical Nutrition is responsible for enteral nutrition and supplements in order to prevent and treat malnutrition in specific target groups. Performance Nutrition deals with all aspects of "functional food" for children, selected groups of adults and the senior population. Nestlé Nutrition Communication is responsible for providing updated information on nutritional issues within and outside the Company. Finally, the medical/scientific group co-ordinates world-wide research and development in the field of nutrition, clinical studies and scientific information, among these the Nestlé Nutrition Workshops.

Since the well-established Nestlé Nutrition Workshop Series was, until now, aimed at infant nutrition only, we decided to organise other workshops aimed towards adult nutrition. The first Nestlé Clinical and Performance Nutrition Workshop took place in October 1997 in Lausanne, Switzerland, and we are pleased to present this first book, of a hopefully long-lasting series, covering the subject of malnutrition.

Prevention and treatment of malnutrition is the important goal in clinical nutrition. The early and precise diagnosis of malnutrition is essential in order to initiate nutritional therapy as soon as possible.

Only during the acute phase of disease are patients kept in hospital, where experts in the field of diagnosis and treatment of malnutrition are available. During the rehabilitation phase, malnourished elderly patients are often treated at home or in nursing homes, where the quality of nutritional support depends on the knowledge of the attending physican or dietician. In elderly persons "without overt disease", low-degree malnutrition is often overlooked and no therapy is offered.

The interactions between malnutrition of the elderly, on the one hand, and altered immunity, increased morbidity and mortality, on the other hand, are well documented. The "Mini Nutritional Assessment" procedure (see Appendix) is a diagnostic tool which can be easily handled by general practitioners, dieticians and nursing personnel. It is not time-consuming and does not require sophisticated equipment to perform.

Therefore, its broad application could assist in the prevention and early treatment of malnutrition and, thus, allow elderly people to benefit from improved health enabling them to take full advantage of their "best years".

Prof. Ferdinand Haschke, MD
Vice-President
Nestec Ltd., Vevey, Switzerland

Mini Nutritional Assessment (MNA): Research and Practice in the Elderly:
B. Vellas; P.J. Garry; Y. Guigoz (eds),
Nestlé Nutrition Workshop Series Clinical & Performance Programme, Vol. 1, pp. 3–12,
Nestec Ltd.; Vevey/S. Karger AG, Basel, © 1999.

The Mini Nutritional Assessment (MNA) for Grading the Nutritional State of Elderly Patients: Presentation of the MNA, History and Validation

Yves Guigoz and Bruno Vellas[a]

Nestlé Research Center, Nestec Ltd., Lausanne, Switzerland;
[a] Department of Internal Medicine and Clinical Gerontology,
CHU Purpan-Casselardit, Toulouse, France

The Mini Nutritional Assessment (MNA), which is composed of simple measurements and brief questions that can be completed in about 10 min, was designed and validated to provide a rapid assessment of the nutritional status of frail elderly people in order to facilitate nutrition intervention [1, 2].

The incidence of protein-energy malnutrition is rather low in people living at home (5–10%). The frail elderly population is, however, at increased risk of malnutrition, and protein-energy malnutrition reaches significant levels in older persons in hospital (20–60%) or who are institutionalized (10–85%; Fig. 1) [2–4]. This goes mainly unrecognized [5], owing to the lack of a specific, validated instrument to detect malnutrition in these elderly persons, and if recognized it is not taken into account (Table 1) [6]. Malnutrition in the elderly has been associated with greater susceptibility to infection, longer stay at hospital, and higher mortality [7, 8].

Use of valid and reliable instruments to assess nutritional status has been absent from most geriatric assessment programs. Simple and rapid screening tests are, however, in use in comprehensive geriatric assessment of cognitive problems, autonomy, gait and balance, and depression [9; see chapter entitled: Comprehensive Geriatric Assessment (CGA) and the MNA: An overview of CGA, Nutritional Assessment and Development of a Shortened Version of the MNA, in this volume]. Rubenstein has reported that the use of well-validated instruments makes geriatric assessment more reliable and easier [9]. Comprehensive nutritional assessment is long and complex, mainly composed of social and clinical history,

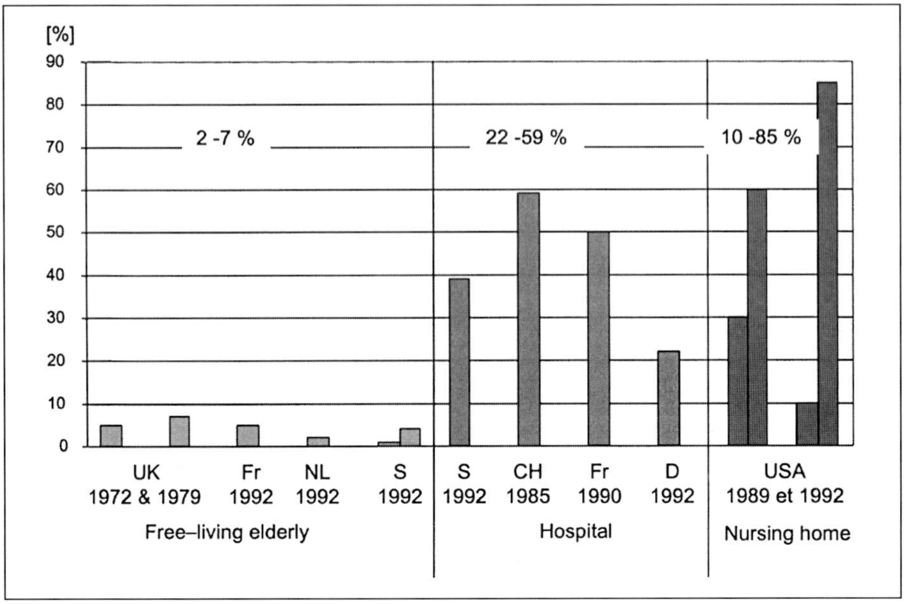

Fig. 1. Prevalence of malnutrition in different elderly groups. UK = United Kingdom; Fr = France; NL = The Netherlands; S = Sweden; CH = Switzerland; D = Germany. (Adapted from Guigoz *et al.*, 1996 [2].)

Table 1. Detection of malnutrition on admission to hospital (n = 121 patients, age 70–98 years)

55%	36%	8%
Malnourished (< 90% of normal weight for height)	Recognized as malnourished on admission	Nutritional support

Adapted from Mowé & Bøhmer [6].

anthropometry, evaluation of dietary intakes, and clinical laboratory analysis [10, 11]. Therefore we decided to design and validate a tool to evaluate the nutritional status of the elderly.

The aim of the MNA is to evaluate the risk of malnutrition in order to permit early nutritional intervention when needed, without necessitating a specialized nutritional assessment team [1, 2]. The following requirements were necessary to obtain a simple and rapid evaluation test: a reliable scale, with definition of thresholds, compatible with the skills of a generalist assessor with minimal bias on behalf of the data collector, acceptable to patients, and inexpensive.

The MNA test (for the MNA form, see Appendix at the end of this volume) is composed of simple measurements and rapid questions so that it can be performed in approximately 10 min or less [1, 2]:

1. Anthropometric measurements (weight, height, and weight loss);
2. Dietary questionnaire (eight questions, related to number of meals, food and fluid intake, and autonomy of feeding);
3. Global assessment (six questions related to lifestyle, medication, and mobility);
4. Subjective assessment (self-perception of health and nutrition).

The scoring of each part allows elderly patients to be classified as: (a) adequately nourished; (b) at risk of malnutrition, and (c) malnourished.

The MNA has been validated on elderly populations (>600 elderly people) ranging in age from 65 to 90 years and above, from the very frail to the very active, in three successive studies [1, 2]: (i) a study on setting up the test in 155 elderly subjects, from very healthy to severely malnourished elderly patients (Toulouse, 1991); (ii) a study on validation and testing of the discriminatory potential of the MNA on 120 elderly subjects, from the frail to the healthy elderly (Toulouse, 1993), and (iii) a complementary validation study in a different cultural context on non-institutionalized elderly people from the New Mexico Aging Process Study [1, 12].

The MNA test was validated using two principal criteria: (i) clinical status – a nutritional assessment done independently by two physicians trained in nutrition, on the basis of the subject's clinical file, without knowledge of MNA results, and (ii) a comprehensive nutritional assessment including measure of the anthropometric markers (height, knee height, weight, body mass index (BMI), and skinfold thickness) according to Chumlea [13, 14], an evaluation of dietary intake (dietary history, three-day food record combined with an interview with frequency checklist of foods) [15], and measurement of biological markers (albumin, prealbumin, transferrin, retinol-binding protein, C-reactive protein, α_1-acid glycoprotein, ceruloplasmin, cholesterol, triglycerides, vitamins A, D, E, B1, B2, B6, and B12, folate, copper, zinc, hematocrit, hemoglobin, and blood cell count) [1].

For this purpose, clinical status was used as the gold standard, and comparisons were done using descriptive statistics, principal component analysis, and discriminant analysis [1]. The specificity of the MNA was performed by cross-classification of the two populations (Toulouse, 1991 and Toulouse, 1993) using the equations from the discriminant analysis. These results showed that for these two studies the MNA without biochemical indices could definitely classify 70–75% of elderly people as normal or undernourished. However, 25–30% of the subjects were situated in a buffer zone between these two classes (normal and undernutrition) and should be classified as at risk of malnutrition (or as borderline). They need further assessment by biochemical indices or clinical evaluation [1].

Finally the threshold values for the MNA scale were set by cross-tabulation of the MNA scores with the serum albumin concentrations (excluding the subjects with inflammation, that is, serum C-reactive protein >20 mg/l) as independent variables. In this way the following threshold values were set for the MNA [1]:

Score (maximum 30 points)	Nutritional status
≥24	Well-nourished / normal
17–23.5	At risk of malnutrition / borderline
<17	Malnourished

The longitudinal study, the New Mexico Aging Process Study [12], examines the nutrition and health status of non-institutionalized elderly people, and represents a healthy aging population with almost 50% aged between 75 and 85 years and more than 10% over 85 years of age. An evaluation of nutritional status using the MNA indicated that even in a healthy elderly group about 20% of the elderly people (60 of 347) are borderline and should be assessed for risk of malnutrition, even if albumin levels and BMI were in the normal range. However, their dietary energy intakes tended to be lower, at 1,833 ± 508 kcal/day (n = 265) for the well-nourished and 1,639 ± 527 kcal/day (n = 51) for the at-risk subjects. These differences were not statistically significant ($p < 0.10$) [1]. These results suggest that the MNA is able to assess nutritional status in the elderly before severe changes in weight or albumin levels occur.

Protein-energy malnutrition appears to be a strong independent risk factor for 1-year postdischarge mortality [8]. One year after nutritional screening with the MNA, the following mortality was observed (Toulouse, 1991): malnourished (MNA score <17) 48%, at risk of malnutrition (MNA score 17–23.5) 24%, well-nourished (MNA score ≥24) 0% [16]. Sensitivity (in this case the ability to detect malnutrition) and specificity (the ability to classify the well-nourished correctly) were calculated for the MNA (Toulouse, 1991), using clinical nutritional status as a reference, and showed a sensitivity of 96% and a specificity of 98% [16]. Figures 2–5 show the good correlation between the MNA and nutritional markers (Toulouse, 1991) such as serum transthyretin (prealbumin; correlation coefficient $r = 0.58$; $p < 0.0001$; n = 147), serum folate ($r = 0.53$; $p < 0.0001$; n = 140), vitamin

Fig. 2. MNA and serum transthyretin (prealbumin) levels (Toulouse, 1991); n = 147 (each dot represents one subject). Normal values: 0.20–0.40 g/l. MNA threshold values: <17 = malnourished; 17–23.5 = at risk of malnutrition; ≥24 = well-nourished. Correlation coefficient, $r = 0.58$ ($p < 0.0001$).

Fig. 3. MNA and serum folate levels (Toulouse, 1991); n = 140 (each dot represents one subject). Normal values: >3 ng/ml (= 6.8 nmol/l). MNA threshold values: <17 = malnourished; 17–23.5 = at risk of malnutrition; ≥24 = well-nourished. Correlation coefficient, $r = 0.53$ ($p < 0.0001$).

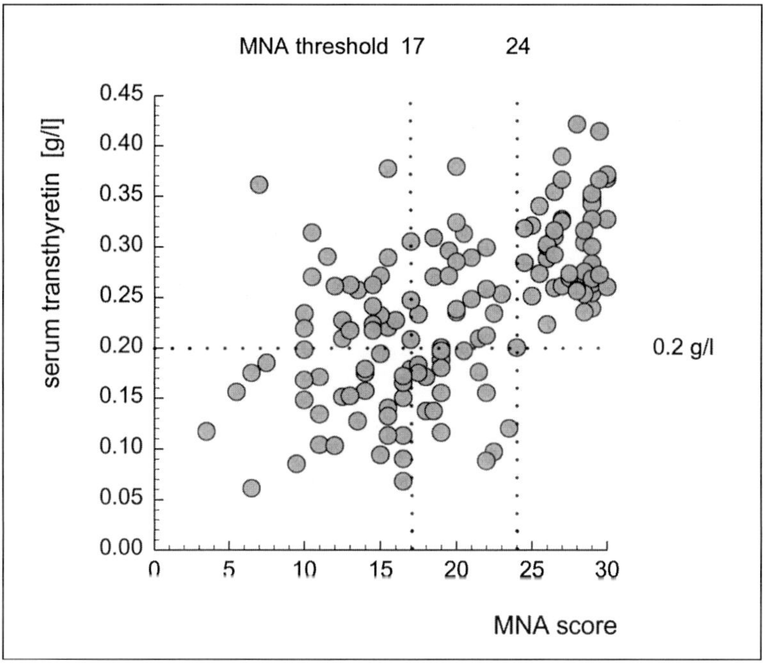
MNA threshold 17
24
serum transthyretin [g/l]
0.45
0.40
0.35
0.30
0.25
0.20
0.15
0.10
0.05
0.00
0.2 g/l
0
5
10
15
20
25
30
MNA score

2

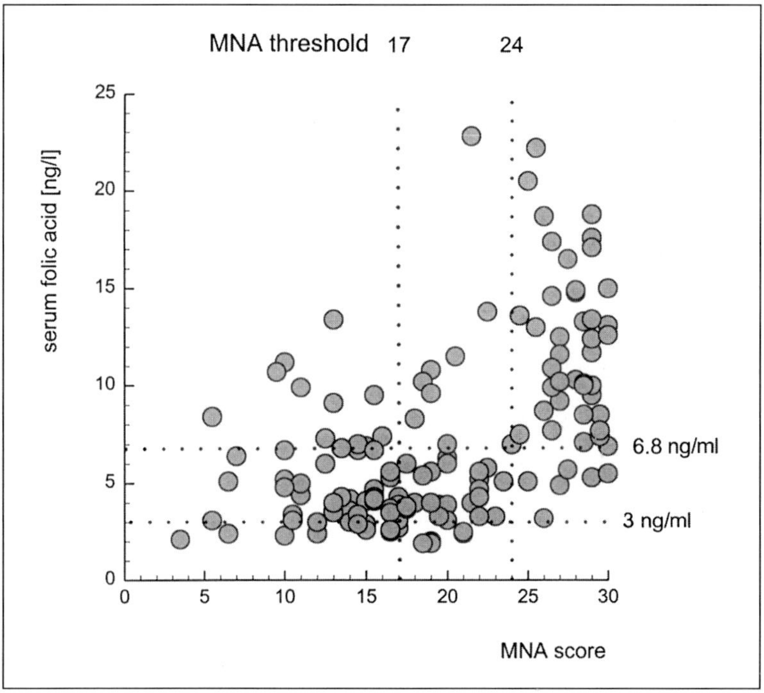
MNA threshold 17
24
serum folic acid [ng/l]
25
20
15
10
5
0
6.8 ng/ml
3 ng/ml
0
5
10
15
20
25
30
MNA score

3

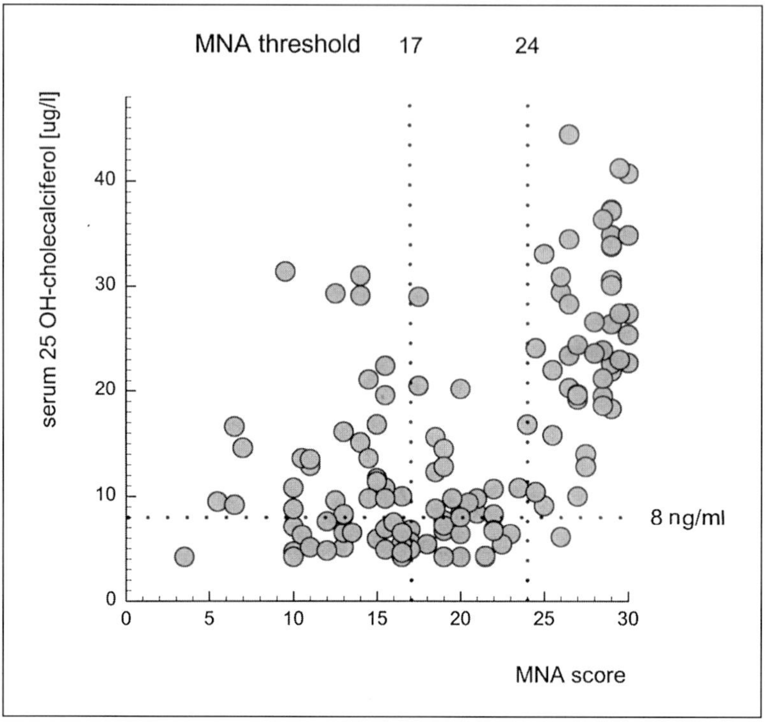

MNA threshold
17
24
serum 25 OH-cholecalciferol [ug/l]
40
30
20
10
0
0
5
10
15
20
25
30
8 ng/ml
MNA score

4

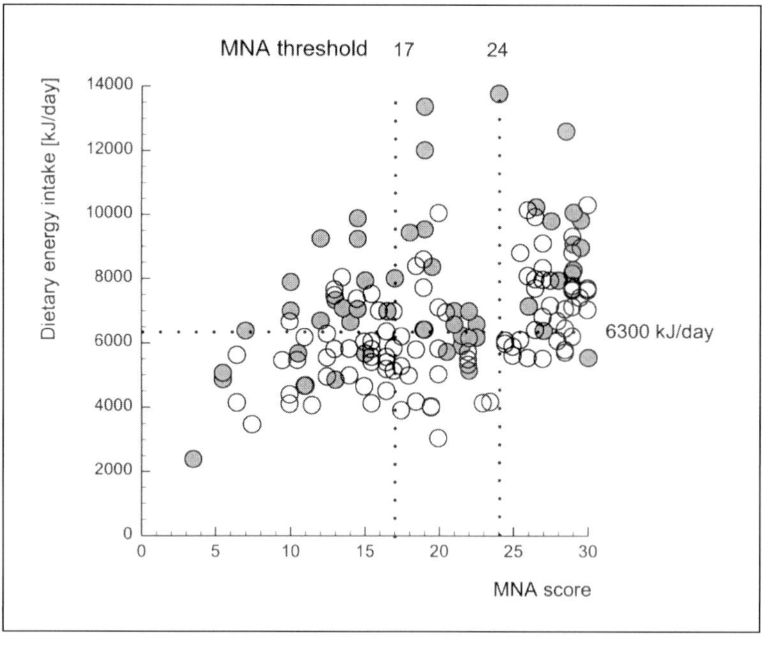

MNA threshold
17
24
Dietary energy intake [kJ/day]
14000
12000
10000
8000
6000
4000
2000
0
0
5
10
15
20
25
30
6300 kJ/day
MNA score

5

D (1-hydroxy-cholecalciferol; $r = 0.53$; $p < 0.0001$; n = 133), and energy intakes ($r = 0.41$; $p < 0.0001$; n = 151). These results indicate the capacity of the MNA to reflect the nutritional status and the risk of malnutrition.

Examples of the identification of nutritional problems using the MNA are given in Table 2 for different situations: living at home, ambulatory care (general

Table 2. Prevalence (%) of malnutrition: MNA screening in different situations

	Well-nourished ≥24	At-risk 17–23.5	Mal-nourished <17	
Albuquerque (n = 356/420)				P. Garry (1995)
Hispanic	72	27	1	
Non-Hispanic white	85	15	0	
Belfast (n = 31)				I.M. Rea (1996)
Free-living, 85–96 years old	44	50	6	
Belgium (n = 72/137)				M. Griep (1995)
Community	97	3	0	
Retirement homes	58	40	2	
Toulouse (n = 91)				S. Lauque (1994)
Nursing home	35	48	27	
Paris (n = 55)				C. Philip-Baudry (1996)
Home care	29	53	18	
Barcelona (n = 87)				A. Salva (1995)
Long-term care	47	47	6	
Mendrisio (n = 166)				P. Quadri (1996)
Admission to hospital	52	33	15	
St Maurice (n = 200)				M. Coutet (1996)
General practitioner	88	12	0	
Nursing home	45	49	6	
Short-term care	28	62	10	
Long-term care	4	66	30	

Fig. 4. MNA and serum vitamin D (25-OH) levels (Toulouse, 1991); n = 133 (each dot represents one subject). Normal values: 8–100 ng/ml. MNA threshold values: <17 = malnourished; 17–23.5 = at risk of malnutrition; ≥24 = well-nourished. Correlation coefficient, $r = 0.53$ ($p < 0.0001$).

Fig. 5. MNA and dietary energy intakes (Toulouse, 1991); n = 151 (each dot represents one subject; men (●) = 50, women (○) = 100). Two thirds of French RDA = 6,300 kJ/day (1,500 kcal/day). MNA threshold values: <17 = malnourished; 17–23.5 = at risk of malnutrition; ≥24 = well-nourished. Correlation coefficient, $r = 0.41$ ($p < 0.0001$).

practitioner or home care), retirement homes, nursing homes and hospitals, including short- and long-term care [17]. The prevalence of malnutrition in free-living elderly people was 0–6%; in nursing homes, 2–27%, and in hospital, 10–30%. These studies show that the MNA is good at discriminating undernourished elderly people and, along with the other chapters in this book, strongly support its value in assessing the nutritional status of elderly people under different conditions.

Conclusions

In summary, the MNA was developed and validated for the early detection of protein-energy malnutrition in the elderly in three successive studies [1, 2]. It fulfills the criteria for nutritional evaluation: sensitivity, specificity, cost, and targeting to a specific group (frail elderly people), as proposed by Rush in his recent review on screening in old people [18]. It has now been translated by specialists into more than 15 languages and is freely available.

The MNA allows physicians and health professionals to make a rapid and reliable evaluation of the nutritional status of elderly patients, to recognize those at risk of nutritional problems.

References

1. Guigoz Y, Vellas B, Garry PJ. Mini Nutritional Assessment: a practical assessment tool for grading the nutritional state of elderly patients. *Facts Res Gerontol* 1994; (suppl 2): 15–60.
2. Guigoz Y, Vellas B, Garry PJ. Assessing the nutritional status of the elderly: the Mini Nutritional Assessment as part of the geriatric evaluation. *Nutr Rev* 1996; 54: S59–65.
3. Rudman D, Feller AG. Protein-calorie undernutrition in the nursing home. *J Am Geriatr Soc* 1989; 37: 173–83.
4. Kerstetter JE, Holhausen BA, Fitz PA. Malnutrition in the institutionalized older adult. *J Am Diet Assoc* 1992; 92: 1109–16.
5. McWhirter JP, Pennington CR. Incidence and recognition of malnutrition in hospital. *BMJ* 1994; 308: 945–8.
6. Mowé M, Bøhmer T. The prevalence of undiagnosed protein-calorie undernutrition of hospitalized elderly patients. *J Am Geriatr Soc* 1991; 39: 1089–92.
7. Michel JP, Lesourd B, Conne P, *et al.* Prevalence of infections and their risk factors in geriatric institutions: a one-day multicentre survey. *WHO Bull* 1991; 69: 35–41.
8. Sullivan DH, Walls RC, Lipschitz DA. Protein-energy undernutrition and the risk of mortality within 1 y of hospital discharge in a select population of geriatric rehabilitation patients. *Am J Clin Nutr* 1991; 53: 599–605.
9. Rubenstein LZ, Bernabei R, Wieland D, eds. *Geriatric assessment technology: state of the art.* Milan: Kurtiz Publishing Co, 1995.
10. Lee RD, Nieman DC, eds. *Nutritional assessment.* Madison, Benchmark Publishers, 1993.
11. Shenkin A, Cederblad G, Isaksson MEB. Laboratory assessment of protein-energy status. *Clin Chim Acta* 1996; 253: S5–59.
12. Garry PJ, Goodwin JS, Hunt WC, *et al.* Nutritional status in a healthy elderly population: dietary and supplemental intake. *Am J Clin Nutr* 1982; 36: 319–31.

13. Chumlea WC, Roche AF, Steinbaugh ML. Anthropometric approaches to the nutritional assessment of the elderly. In: Munro HN, Danford DE, eds. *Nutrition, aging, and the elderly.* New York: Plenum Press, 1989: 335–61.
14. Guo S, Wu X, Vellas B, Guigoz Y, Chumlea WC. Prediction of stature in the French elderly. *Age Nutr* 1994; 5: 169.
15. De Groot CPGM, van Staveren WA. *Nutrition and the elderly.* A European collaborative study in cooperation with the World Health Organisation, Special Programme for Research on Aging (WHO-SPRA), and the International Union of Nutritional Sciences Committee on Geriatric Nutrition. Manual of Operations. Wageningen: Euronut Report 11, 1988.
16. Guigoz Y, Vellas B. Test d'évaluation de l'état nutritionnel de la personne agée: le Mini Nutritional Assessment (MNA). *Med Hyg* 1995; 53: 1965–9.
17. Guigoz Y, Nourashemi F, Vellas B. The MNA (Mini Nutritional Assessment): update. *Facts, research and intervention in geriatrics.* Paris: Serdi Publishing Co, 1997: 105–12.
18. Rush D. Nutrition screening in old people: its place in a coherent practice of preventive health care. *Annu Rev Nutr* 1997; 17: 101–25.

Discussion

Dr. Cohendy: I would like to ask about frail elderly patients. Have you found any relation between the MNA score and the level of hemoglobin, hematocrit or iron?

Dr. Guigoz: We didn't look at iron. There was, however, a relation between MNA score and hemoglobin and hematocrit in the first Toulouse study.

Dr. Cohendy: Is this relation sufficiently strong to predict anemia or a problem related to anemia in elderly people?

Dr. Guigoz: This should be looked at; we have not done so.

Dr. Rubenstein: The fact that people are now looking at nutrition as part of geriatric assessment is really important, but when you described the ongoing use of MNA, most of it seems to be related to research databases or longitudinal population studies. Approximately how many places in the world are now using this assessment as a clinical tool in day-to-day practice? Do you have any feeling for that?

Dr. Vellas: I don't know – most people who use the score probably don't go to meetings! However, in the Toulouse area we are now seeing more and more patients with MNA scores done by the family practitioner, so it seems to be fairly widespread.

Dr. Guigoz: In Geneva, every patient coming to the geriatric hospital has an MNA score.

Dr. Vellas: We are also receiving increasing numbers of papers submitted for publication from geriatric hospitals where the MNA is in use.

Dr. Morley: In our hospital, both in the outpatients and in subacute care, our fellows have started to use MNA spontaneously, so it is a user-friendly instrument. We did not ask them to do it. They introduced it themselves. This tells us that it is an enjoyable instrument for people who are not used to assessing nutrition, and this is a positive feature.

Although we did not specifically look at the question of the frail obese population, I believe that the MNA probably does pick up malnutrition in obese people who are running into trouble. It seems capable of looking at both ends of the spectrum, and that is one of the positive aspects of the MNA. We must remember that it has high sensitivity, but lower specificity. That's fine for a screening tool – if you make it too specific, you will miss too many people at risk. The purpose of this tool, which can be used by anyone, is to make sure that people are referred for more sophisticated workup.

I was wondering if you have data from the Toulouse study on hospital admissions and deaths occurring in people who have had MNA. Have you looked to see if the MNA is predictive in that population, or in the New Mexico population?

Dr. Vellas: We do have a correlation between MNA and mortality, but we have not collected retrospective data.

I have a comment relating to Dr. Rubenstein's question. When medical students come to do geriatric medicine, they like to learn things that they don't learn in other departments. They can learn how to treat pneumonia or hypertension in most departments. When they come to the geriatric department, they like to learn how to use a tool such as MNA. When students have learned how to use MNA, they will use it more and more.

Dr. Berner: With regard to obesity, the only existing data on obesity as a risk factor come from the Metropolitan Life Tables, where one can see flattening of the J-shaped curve with aging up to a horizontal line above 80. Therefore MNA is very important in obese elderly people where borderline nutritional deficiency may be present but masked by their obesity.

Dr. Rossle: You say that the MNA has been translated into about 20 languages, and has been validated in France and the USA. Would you recommend it for use with people of any ethnic origin? Do you think there are any limitations for the use of this tool?

Dr. Guigoz: I don't think so. It is validated for elderly people so it should be suitable for any elderly person, though maybe we should check the anthropometric values for different populations. We used the Toulouse population as the standard, but it is possible that other populations may need different anthropometric standards.

Mini Nutritional Assessment (MNA): Research and Practice in the Elderly:
B. Vellas; P.J. Garry; Y. Guigoz (eds),
Nestlé Nutrition Workshop Series Clinical & Performance Programme, Vol. 1, pp. 13–22,
Nestec Ltd.; Vevey/S. Karger AG, Basel, © 1999.

The Mini Nutritional Assessment and Body Composition in Healthy Adults

Wm. Cameron Chumlea, Gwendolyn Hall, Flavius Lilly,
R.M. Siervogel and Shumei S. Guo

*Division of Human Biology, Department of Community Health,
Wright State University School of Medicine, Dayton, Ohio, USA*

The normal physiological consequences of aging alter body size and composition. These alterations affect or are affected by weight-related health conditions and nutritional status. Elderly persons who lose body weight are reported to have a lower survival rate than those who gain weight or remain stable [1, 2]. A loss of weight also reduces levels of functional activity, is associated with depressed immune function and increases the risk of morbidity and mortality [3]. Following a severe illness, normal physiological function is not regained until weight and body composition are restored to their pre-illness levels [3]. There is also the effect of sarcopenia or a loss of muscle tissue with age upon body strength, gait, and balance, which increases the risk of falls and subsequent injury [4, 5]. These changes in weight and body composition, if severe or of a sufficient duration during illness, can exacerbate the outcomes of chronic disease and increase the risk for infirmity or physical disability [4, 6]. The overall impact of these changes in body composition can be a decline in function and a decline in health status.

Assessing nutritional status in the elderly is critical for determining and maintaining health status. Poor nutritional status in the elderly is related to the increased risk of morbidity, and frank malnutrition is associated with an increased incidence of morbidity and mortality [7, 8]. In addition, nutritional status, which is reflected in body composition, is related to the overall quality of life and health and the demand for and cost of health services [9–12]. These relations are well recognized, but often poorly addressed because of the lack or limited availability of suitable screening techniques and methods of assessing nutritional status. Laboratory and clinical methods are available, but may not be appropriate in some nonclinical settings or are associated with high costs that may limit insurance or government health service payment.

In the United States, the assessment of nutritional status of the elderly has a distinct role in the application of managed care to health services for the elderly. This assessment role is similar to that used to assess mental, cognitive, and functional status by the several standardized tests available for these conditions [13]. Attempts by some at screening for or indexing nutritional status have been directed at the general population or specifically at hospital inpatients [10, 14–16]. Screening the nutritional status of hospital and surgical patients for risk of complications can lead to improvements in the management and care of these individuals. At the same time, increasing the elderly public's awareness of its nutritional condition is an important part of public health [17]. However, some of the screening tools or indices are not adequate for identifying the elderly person who, while supposedly well-nourished, is at risk of becoming malnourished [16].

The Mini Nutritional Assessment (MNA) is a practical, noninvasive technique for rapidly evaluating the potential risk of malnutrition among elderly persons in clinics, at home, or in nursing homes by health care professionals as a part of regular care or for acute and chronic conditions [13, 17, 18]. The MNA has received recognition as a suitable screening tool and has been validated to a limited degree in samples of elderly persons from several countries [19, 20]. However, the relation of MNA scores to actual measures of body stores of muscle and adipose tissue or body composition has not been addressed. The present report looks at the association of MNA scores in healthy adults to their measured levels of body composition, that is, fat-free mass (FFM), total body fat (TBF), and percent body fat (%BF). If the MNA is to be a useful nutritional assessment screening tool, then MNA scores should bear, to some degree, a real relation with the amounts of these body components, regardless of a person's age.

Methods

Our study sample included 24 men and 37 women, 20–78 years of age. These were healthy, free-living persons who were participants in Health Assessment 2000, a National Institutes of Health funded study of multifrequency bioelectrical impedance at Wright State University School of Medicine. The MNA was administered by a trained health researcher, and the participant's answers recorded into a laptop computer. Details of the MNA, development of its scoring system, and validation have been reported [13]. Anthropometry was collected using methods similar to those used in the National Health and Nutrition Examination Surveys [21]. Individual values for body composition (FFM, TBF, and %BF) were ob-

Table 1. Univariate statistics for men for body composition, anthropometric, and laboratory variables by Mini Nutritional Assessment (MNA) classification

Variable	Men (n = 6) with MNA <24				Men (n = 19) with MNA ≥24			
	Mean	SD	Min	Max	Mean	SD	Min	Max
MNA score	22.7	0.4	22.0	23.0	27.8	1.3	24.5	29.5
Age, years	45.7	15.8	24.6	58.5	52.8	15.7	20.9	77.7
Stature, cm	181.5	6.4	176.6	194.1	179.1	7.0	163.6	194.9
Weight, kg	88.5	14.4	76.7	114.8	86.0	13.5	58.7	115.8
FFM, kg	64.5	6.1	59.3	75.6	63.6	10.3	41.4	82.3
%BF	26.3	7.9	16.6	34.4	26.1	7.3	8.5	38.9
TBF, kg	23.9	10.0	13.4	37.3	22.7	7.7	6.9	41.5
BMI, kg/m^2	27.1	5.5	21.5	36.8	26.7	3.1	19.9	34.9
Arm circ, cm	34.7	5.0	29.4	44.0	34.6	3.4	29.4	44.1
Calf circ, cm	39.4	2.9	35.9	43.7	38.7	2.8	31.3	42.9
Hemoglobin, g/dl	14.9	1.0	13.6	16.5	14.7	1.3	10.5	16.6
Hematocrit, %	42.4	3.0	37.9	46.0	42.0	3.5	30.5	46.4
Cholesterol, mg/dl	209.0	15.9	195.0	237.0	197.6	34.8	131.0	296.0
Triglyceride, mg/dl	189.8	88.4	82.0	282.0	181.1	144.6	24.0	606.0

tained from dual energy X-ray absorptiometry (DXA) scans using a Lunar DPX machine with 3.6z software [22]. Laboratory values for hemoglobin, hematocrit, total cholesterol, and triglycerides were determined at a local certified laboratory. Fasting blood was not drawn. All procedures were approved by the Institutional Review Board of Wright State University.

Results

In this sample, the men, on average, were significantly ($p < 0.05$) taller, heavier, and had a greater FFM than the women, who had greater TBF and a higher %BF than the men. There were six men and four women with MNA scores between 20 and 23, placing them within the proposed range for "at risk" of malnutrition (17 to <24). The remainder of the sample (19 men and 32 women) had MNA scores between 24 and 30, indicating that they were "well-nourished" according to the scoring criteria established for the MNA [13]. The univariate statistics for the measured variables in the at-risk and well-nourished groups of men and women are presented in Tables 1 and 2, respectively.

In the at-risk groups of men and women, there were no distinguishing characteristics among the measured variables that were significant when compared with corresponding values in the well-nourished groups. The means for FFM, TBF,

Table 2. Univariate statistics for women for body composition, anthropometric and laboratory variables by Mini Nutritional Assessment (MNA) classification

Variable	Women (n = 4) with MNA <24				Women (n = 32) with MNA ≥24			
	Mean	SD	Min	Max	Mean	SD	Min	Max
MNA score	21.1	1.4	20.0	23.0	26.7	1.5	24.0	30.0
Age, years	58.4	10.2	43.8	67.9	59.1	13.1	19.9	76.0
Stature, cm	164.5	6.8	157.0	170.9	162.0	5.2	151.0	174.4
Weight, kg	72.6	14.5	58.0	90.0	71.2	12.5	48.7	95.5
FFM, kg	43.7	2.8	40.7	46.5	42.7	4.8	34.5	52.9
%BF	38.9	9.0	28.1	49.5	39.9	6.9	22.7	50.0
TBF, kg	29.5	12.3	16.4	44.7	29.4	9.1	13.7	47.7
BMI, kg/m^2	27.2	7.6	19.9	36.5	27.2	4.9	19.1	37.7
Arm circ, cm	33.3	5.7	27.9	40.2	32.6	4.1	24.1	42.1
Calf circ, cm	39.9	5.4	34.7	46.8	36.6	2.7	30.9	42.5
Hemoglobin, g/dl	13.5	0.8	12.7	14.5	13.4	0.9	11.6	16.6
Hematocrit, %	37.5	2.7	34.8	40.1	38.9	2.3	35.7	47.5
Cholesterol, mg/dl	226.3	31.2	202.0	269.0	229.6	40.5	157.0	310.0
Triglyceride, mg/dl	149.3	37.4	99.0	189.0	163.3	103.6	24.0	391.0

and %BF of the at-risk groups of men and women were similar to those of the well-nourished groups. This was also true for the other measured or calculated variables (Tables 1 and 2). Some men and women in the at-risk groups were obese in terms of body composition values for FFM, TBF, %BF, and body mass index (BMI, kg/m^2). At the same time, there were men and women in the well-nourished group who had low levels of body fatness.

All the participants were also given the MOS 36-item short-form health survey (SF-36) to assess their levels of health and physical function, both of which were high [23]. When the SF-36 scores for the eight health status scales or components were divided between the at-risk and well-nourished groups of men and women, there were again no distinguishing intergroup differences (Table 3). A high component score is an indication that an individual is performing a high level in that component and has no problems related to the performance of that component [23]. For some of the components, the SF-36 scores were slightly lower in the at-risk groups than in the well-nourished groups, such as for bodily pain and general health in the men, physical function and social function in the women, and for mental health in both the men and women. Among other SF-36 component scores, such as for vitality, the at-risk groups had slightly higher scores than the well-nourished groups.

To determine if there were specific questions in the MNA that were categorizing well-nourished or even obese individuals as at risk of malnutrition, we compared the answer to the individual MNA questions between the at-risk and well-

Table 3. SF-36 mean component health status scores in the well-nourished and at-risk groups

	Well-nourished	At-risk
Men		
Bodily pain	49.47	46.66
Physical functioning	91.05	96.6
Role physical	94.7	100.0
General health	80.0	75.16
Vitality	70.26	75.0
Social functioning	91.44	97.9
Role emotional	94.7	100.0
Mental health	86.15	82.0
Women		
Bodily pain	52.18	55.0
Physical functioning	81.87	73.75
Role physical	82.03	75.0
General health	75.5	79.75
Vitality	61.87	65.0
Social functioning	88.67	75.0
Role emotional	77.08	100.0
Mental health	79.62	75.0

Table 4. Comparison of MNA answers by questions

Questions	d.f.	χ^2	Probability
Recent weight loss	2	9.687	0.008
More than three prescription drugs a day	1	1.608	0.205
Psychological stress or acute disease in the past 3 months	1	9.241	0.002
How many full meals do you eat each day?	2	4.100	0.129
One serving of dairy products each day	2	1.876	0.391
Two or more servings of beans or eggs per week			
A serving of meat, fish, or poultry each day			
Two or more servings of fruits or vegetables each day	1	6.600	0.010
Food intake declined over the past 3 months	1	0.114	0.735
How much fluid do you drink each day?	2	0.649	0.723
Do you think that you have any nutritional problems?	1	1.724	0.189
How do you consider your health status?	2	0.902	0.637

nourished groups (Table 4). A χ^2 analysis found significant ($p < 0.05$) group differences for only three of the MNA questions: recent weight loss; recent psychological stress or acute disease, and servings of fruit and vegetables. These were the only questions that distinguished the answers of the at-risk groups from those of the well-nourished groups.

Discussion

In the at-risk groups, the ages of the four women were between 40 and 70 years, 2 of the men were younger than 40 years, and the remaining four men were between 50 and 60 years of age. Means for measures of FFM, TBF, %BF, and arm and calf circumferences and for calculated values of BMI for the 10 men and women at risk of malnutrition were not different from corresponding means for the 51 well-nourished men and women. Thus approximately 16% of the present sample were identified as at risk for malnutrition, but their levels of body composition and laboratory blood values were similar or fell within the range of those in the sample identified as well-nourished. Values for albumin were not measured.

Our findings indicate that the current version of the MNA may have some limitations in its sensitivity and specificity in relation to measured values for body composition, owing to this apparent categorization of some healthy individuals as at risk for malnutrition. In general, there was nothing identifiable about the at-risk group that indicated why they were classified in this manner by the MNA. In fact, some of the at-risk men and women were clearly obese and some of the well-nourished group were thin. Some of the men and women in the at-risk group had high BMI values, well above 27 which is considered a cutoff point for obesity. These same individuals had %BFs of 35% to 50%. In addition, some of the at-risk men and women had low BMI values of 19 to 21, as did members of the well-nourished group. There is much justifiable concern regarding low levels of BMI, FFM and sarcopenia among the elderly [24]. At the same time, obesity is also common among the elderly [25–27].

High and low values of BMI are associated with increased risks of disease, and the relation of BMI with all cause mortality is reportedly U-shaped [28]. Mortality associated with low BMI consists of tuberculosis, obstructive lung disease, and lung and stomach cancer. The mortality associated with high BMI is cerebrovascular and cardiovascular disease, diabetes, and colon cancer. Using a cutoff definition for risk of overweight or underweight based on adequacy of BMI, one can map the prevalence of overweight and underweight conditions. However, the cutoff points for centiles as markers for obesity or undernutrition are not clearly established at any age. High and low levels of BMI have been reported to be associated with poor health (medical, psychological, and sociological factors) among the elderly [29]. If BMI is to be used as a marker in the elderly, it should be noted that it is influenced by declining bone mass and changes in hydration of the fat-free body with age; as such, this may limit its value.

Some of the SF-36 components or questions are similar to questions on the MNA that relate to perceived health and emotional and psychological stress. However, there was no apparent trend among the SF-36 health status scores that identified the MNA at-risk groups. When we looked at individual MNA questions, there were three with significant group differences. More people in the at-risk group had lost weight recently than in the well-nourished group. A loss of weight is an indicator of poor nutritional status. However, it is most likely that in these healthy individuals a loss of weight was due to voluntary dieting. This sample was self-selected and could be biased by the inclusion of health-conscious persons who were very interested in their body composition. It may be important to qualify this question to identify individuals on diets or exercise programs.

The second question related to a recent acute illness or psychological stress. This question may be misinterpreted. Obviously, dieting is a psychological stress, and an acute illness could be a cold, sore throat, or flu. It may be important to qualify this question to identify the length of the acute illness, amount of bed rest, length of recovery, or severity or classification of the psychological stress such as loss of a spouse.

The third question related to servings of fruits and vegetables. The answer to this question can be seasonably affected, but most probably reflects possible dieting or lifelong food habits or preferences. There could also be some confusion as to what is a fruit or a vegetable. Potatoes are a vegetable, but are servings of French fries important? Instead, do we want to know about the servings of green leafy vegetables? Surprisingly, the answer to the number of meals per day among these two groups was not different, so the possible dieters were not skipping meals. Since the MNA is used in numerous different cultures, this could be a culturally specific question or one related to lifestyle.

Some other issues to consider as possible questions or qualifiers to the MNA are the level of physical activity, smoking status, socioeconomic level, and type of health care provider. In the USA, a low socioeconomic status and Medicare can explain many apparent race, ethnic, and nutritional differences among groups across the population. A low socioeconomic status is an indicator of possible poor health status and level of care. An additional question concerns the validity of the MNA. To what type of elderly individual person and under what kind of setting should the MNA be administered? There are already clear cases where the MNA has been validated in nursing home and hospital-bound elderly [13, 17]. Should the MNA be used by dietitians monitoring healthy, free-living elderly in retirement villages? How is the MNA to be used for assessing the nutritional status of home-bound, inner city elderly persons of color? Is there a younger age limit to the MNA?

Conclusion

Body composition is an interdependent, multifaceted quantity that is directly related to health and nutritional status. We are capable of determining when the amount or level of FFM starts to decrease or when the distribution of tissues in the body's composition shifts toward a greater than normal level of fat or adipose tissue. In an individual with these conditions, the risk for disease and early death increases, but the magnitude of the changes relative to the threshold for the increased risk is affected by the age, sex, race, living habits, and nutritional status. The MNA is an accepted screening method for classifying the nutritional status or risk of malnutrition (undernutrition) of elderly individuals. The comparison of the MNA scores with concurrent levels of body composition in this study indicates that the MNA does not clearly discriminate differences among all individuals in terms of levels of FFM or body fatness. To clarify these levels in relation to under- or overnutrition, additional studies are recommended to increase the sensitivity and specificity of the MNA in relation to measured values of body stores of fat and protein. Such studies should include state-of-the-art body composition techniques in combination with anthropometry and biochemical measures as defined outcomes. In addition, consideration should be given to the ability of the MNA to detect changes in nutritional status over time. Health care professionals will not just use the MNA once, but will repeat it on the same individuals. How should these repeated assessments be interpreted in relation to real changes in body composition and nutritional status?

Acknowledgments

This work was supported by grants HL53404, HD27063 and HD12252 from the National Institutes of Health, Bethesda, MD.

References

1. Chumlea WC, Guo SS, Cockram DB, Siervogel RM. Mechanical and physiologic modifiers and bioelectrical impedance spectrum determinants of body composition. *Am J Clin Nutr* 1996; 64: 413–22S.
2. Chumlea WC, Guo SS, Glaser RM, Vellas BJ. Sarcopenia, function and health. *J Nutr Health Aging* 1997; 1: 7–12.
3. Dwyer JT, Coleman KA, Krall E, *et al.* Changes in relative weight among institutionalized elderly adults. *J Gerontol* 1987; 42: 246–51.
4. Egbert AM. The dwindles: failure to thrive in older patients. *Nutr Rev* 1996; 54: S525–30.
5. Ettinger WH, Fried LP, Harris T, Shemanski L, Schulz R, Robbins J. Self-reported causes of physical disability in older people: the Cardiovascular Health Study. *J Am Geriatr Soc* 1994; 42: 1035–44.
6. Fasiant C, Lauque S, Guigoz Y, Ghisolfi-Marque A, Vellas BJ, Albarede JL. Nutrition assessment and MNA (Mini Nutritional Assessment). *Facts Res Gerontol* 1995; (suppl: Nutrition): 157–61.
7. Fiatarone MA, Oneill EF, Ryan ND, *et al.* Exercise training and nutritional supplementation for physical frailty in very elderly people. *N Engl J Med* 1994; 330: 1769–75.
8. Guigoz Y, Vellas BJ, Garry PJ. Mini Nutritional Assessment: a practical assessment tool for grading the nutritional state of elderly patients. *Facts Res Gerontol* 1994; 4: 15–59.
9. Guigoz Y, Vellas B, Garry PJ. Assessing the nutritional status of the elderly: the mini nutritional assessment as part of the geriatric evaluation. *Nutr Rev* 1996; 54: S59–65.
10. Harris T, Cook EF, Garrison R, Higgins M, Kannel W, Goldman L. Body mass index and mortality among nonsmoking older persons. The Framingham Heart Study. *JAMA* 1988; 259: 1520–4.
11. Jensen E, Dehlin O, Hagberg B, Samuelsson G, Svensson T. Body mass index in relation to medical, psychological and sociological factors in an 80 year old population. *Facts Res Gerontol* 1995; (suppl: Nutrition): 143–56.
12. Lipschitz DA. Malnutrition in the elderly. *Semin Dermatol* 1991; 10: 273–81.

13. Lipschitz DA, Ham RJ, White JV. An approach to nutrition screening for older Americans. *Am Fam Physician* 1992; 45: 601–8.
14. Lohman TG, Roche AF, Martorell R, eds. *Anthropometric standardization reference manual.* Champaign, IL: Human Kinetics Publishers, 1988.
15. Morley JE. Nutrition assessment is a key component of geriatric assessment. *Facts Res Gerontol* 1994; S2: 5–9.
16. Naber TH, de Bree A, Schermer TR, *et al.* Specificity of indexes of malnutrition when applied to apparently healthy people: the effect of age. *Am J Clin Nutr* 1997; 65: 1721–5.
17. Nikolaus T, Bach M, Siezen S, Oster P, Schlierf G. Assessment of nutritional risk in the elderly. *Ann Nutr Metab* 1995; 39: 340–5.
18. Pertoldi W, Fragiacomo C, Rapin CH, Guigoz Y, Quadri P. The Mini Nutritional Assessment: a predictor of hospital costs in geriatric patients. *J Am Geriatr Soc* 1996; 44: 230.
19. Potter JF, Schafer DF, Bohi RL. In-hospital mortality as a function of body mass index: an age-dependent variable. *J Gerontol* 1988; 43: M59.
20. Roubenoff R, Keyhayias JJ, Dawson-Hughes B, Heymsfield SB. Use of dual-energy X-ray absorptiometry in body composition studies: not yet a "gold standard." *Am J Clin Nutr* 1993; 58: 589–91.
21. Salom IL. Weight control and nutrition: knowing when to intervene. *Geriatrics* 1997; 52: 33–4.
22. Salva A, Bolibar I, Munnoz M, Sacristan V. Results of the "Mini Nutritional Assessment" (MNA) in nursing home residents. *J Am Geriatr Soc* 1996; 44: 11.
23. Seim HC, Holtmeier KB. Treatment of obesity in the elderly. *Am Fam Physician* 1993; 47: 1183–9.
24. Tayback M, Kumanyika S, Chee E. Body weight as a risk factor in the elderly. *Arch Intern Med* 1990; 150: 1065–72.
25. Vellas B, Baumgartner RN, Wayne SJ, *et al.* Relationship between malnutrition and falls in the elderly. *Nutrition* 1992; 8: 105–8.
26. Vellas B, Garry PJ, Albarede JL. Nutritional assessment as part of the geriatric evaluation – the Mini Nutritional Assessment. *Facts Res Gerontol* 1994; S2: 11–13.
27. Wahlqvist ML, Savige GS, Lukito W. Nutritional disorders in the elderly. *Med J Aust* 1995; 163: 376–81.
28. Ware JE, Sherbourne CD. The MOS 36-item short-form health survey (SF-36). *Med Care* 1992; 30: 473–83.
29. White JV. Risk factors for poor nutritional status in older Americans. *Am Fam Physician* 1991; 44: 2087–97.

Discussion

Dr. Morley: When you looked at body composition, particularly in the people who may be losing weight, did you try to correct for the discrepancies in mid-body circumference by using a fat control in the population?

Dr. Chumlea: No, those were just the absolute DXA values.

Dr. Vanderbroele: As I understand it, MNA is validated for elderly people, but the range of your patients was 20–78 years according to your slides. What is the value of doing the analysis in younger people with an instrument that has been validated in elderly people?

Dr. Chumlea: The point I was making is that if the MNA is to be used to identify people who are well nourished, then in a sample that *is* well nourished, it should not misidentify anybody as being at risk. Within this sample, however, it identified 16% of the healthy population as being at risk from malnutrition, so we were looking for reasons why this group was identified. It would appear that this may relate to dieting and to misinterpretation of questions. If we have a potential error of 16% in a sample of elderly people, the number of false-positives will be substantial.

Dr. Morley: I think that you may be wrong in saying that people who are dieting are healthy. A study of ours in the *American Journal of Medicine* [1] shows that one of the commonest presentations of malnutrition in middle-aged people is a therapeutic diet. Therefore it would be good if the MNA picked up dieting people as being at risk. Most physicians assume that if you put somebody on a weight-reducing or low-cholesterol diet, that is good for them. But some people take this to excess, so I don't think it is necessarily bad that dieting shows up positive. All studies will have false-positives, but you need to be aware of those.

Dr. Miller: There was also some work from Seattle in elderly people who lost weight on purpose: they had an excess mortality compared with those who did not [2]. I think this is potentially a dangerous practice in older people. In our population of African-Americans we have many obese people, but I'm unhappy about trying to get them to lose weight, because we don't know what the effects may be. I wonder to what extent we need to differentiate between evaluating *status* – that is, where they are now – and *risk* – where they're headed. I'm using a slightly different term to what you've been talking about here. Maybe one thing that we need to be doing in MNA is to try to see how well it predicts future problems.

Dr. Chumlea: You obviously want to know the person's status at a particular point in time, which gives you specific information, and it may also be that MNA scores are predictive of morbidity or mortality at some point in the future, depending upon age and other factors. So yes, it would be definitely nice to have a measure of current status that has predictive value as well; this could then be used clinically to make further adjustments to dietary management.

Dr. Vellas: Do you have any data on MNA scores in obese people?

Dr. Chumlea: In our sample there were people who had MNA scores below 23 and had 50% body fat. It's worth remembering that an elderly person with muscle wasting who maintains body fat unchanged is effectively becoming obese. People with normal body weight but low muscle mass and a high percentage of body fat may be as much at risk of other nutritional and health problems as frankly obese people.

Dr. Guesry: Don't you think there is probably an age threshold for obesity as a risk factor? You mentioned that it ranks No. 5, but I suppose that it is in adults of around 60–65 years of age. In 80-year-old people obesity may no longer be a risk factor.

Dr. Chumlea: Probably not, except for the matter of physical activity levels. The overweight old person may have more muscle wasting because of reduced activity, which could be harmful.

References

1. Wilson MMG, Vaswani S, Liu D, Morley JE, Miller DK. Prevalence and causes of undernutrition in medical outpatients. *Am J Med* 1998; 104 (1): 56–63.
2. Wallace JI, Schwartz RS, LaCroix AZ, Uhlmann RF, Pearlman RA. Involuntary weight loss in older outpatients: incidence and clinical significance. *J Am Geriatr Soc* 1995; 43: 329–37.

Mini Nutritional Assessment (MNA): Research and Practice in the Elderly:
B. Vellas; P.J. Garry; Y. Guigoz (eds),
Nestlé Nutrition Workshop Series Clinical & Performance Programme, Vol. 1, pp. 23–34,
Nestec Ltd.; Vevey/S. Karger AG, Basel, © 1999.

MNA and Immunity: Nutritional Status and Immunological Markers in the Elderly

E.J. Schiffrin, Yves Guigoz, Geneviève Perruisseau,
Stéphanie Blum, Yves Delneste, Robert Mansourian,
B. Vellas[a] and A. Blancher[a]

Nestlé Research Centre, Nestec Ltd., Lausanne, Switzerland;
[a] Department of Internal Medicine and Laboratory of Immunology,
Pavillon Ch. Lefevre, CHU Purpan-Casselardit, Toulouse, France

An altered (impaired) immune response has previously been detected in elderly individuals [1, 2]. Several investigators have suggested that this impaired immune function is caused by a basic defect in receptor signalling of immune cells and an altered capacity to respond to antigen-dependent activation signals [3].

In fact, any immune response implies the activation and expansion (proliferation) of antigen-specific cells, and it has been reported that with aging a smaller number of immune cells enters into the cell cycle upon antigen or mitogen stimulation [3]. Indeed the ability to produce antibodies and undergo T cell proliferation has become the paradigm of an impaired immune responsiveness with age [4]. Two major mechanisms could be responsible for this observation: (i) a different distribution of lymphocyte subsets with the aging process owing to an abnormal lymphopoietic function, including cellular maturation, and (ii) an intrinsic cellular deficiency resulting in an abnormal response to activation signals. A major participant in T cell activation and proliferation is the interleukin (IL)-2 pathway, which involves the production of IL-2 and IL-2 receptor (IL-2R) expression at the cell surface.

The impaired immune response present in elderly people may be associated with the normal aging process, with chronic pathological conditions, or with malnutrition. Malnutrition is a rather frequent finding in the elderly population (15–60%) in hospitals or living in nursing homes [5]. Therefore the early detection of malnutrition and its correction could be a useful means of preventing intercurrent and terminal infectious events in the aging population.

The Mini Nutritional Assessment (MNA) is a valuable recently developed tool to assess the risk of malnutrition in the elderly [5]. Our aim in this study was to determine whether there is a correlation between the MNA score, other nutritional markers, and defined immunologic indices in the elderly. These immunologic variables included the assessment of major peripheral blood lymphocyte subsets, and the capacity to respond *in vitro* to polyclonal mitogenic stimulation.

Materials and Methods

Subjects

Eighty-eight nursing home patients were classified according to the MNA score into three groups: group 1 (MNA $\geq$24, adequate nutritional status); group 2 (MNA between 17 and 23.5, at risk of malnutrition), and group 3 (MNA score <17, frank malnutrition). Seventy-nine patients completed the immunological study, which took place in Toulouse (Centre de Médecine Gériatrique).

The patients were also grouped according to two other criteria: (i) plasma albumin concentrations, and (ii) the presence of anemia. Based on the first of these criteria, three groups were defined: patients with plasma albumin concentrations of <35 g/l; patients with values between 35 and 40 g/l, and a third group with values of >40 g/l. These albumin ranges were established according to previous nutritional studies [6].

Anemia was defined as a hemoglobin concentration of <12 g/dl for females and <13 g/dl for males [7]. Hematological determinations included total and differential leukocyte count and hematocrit.

Determination of Serum Immunoglobulins

Immunoglobulin isotype (IgG, IgM, IgA) determination was performed by nephelometry (ARRAY 360, Beckman).

Lymphocyte Subsets in Peripheral Blood

Blood samples were collected in sterile EDTA blood collection tubes, and flow cytometric analysis of human leukocyte subsets was performed. A one-step staining procedure was performed with FITC-labeled monoclonal antibodies against T cells (CD3+), B cells (CD19), helper T (CD4+), and suppressor/cytotoxic T cells (CD8+; Immunotech).

The proportion of CD45-RO and CD45-RA subsets within the CD4+ lymphocyte subpopulation was determined by double-staining techniques in flow cytometry (Beckton Dickinson).

In vitro *Lymphocyte Functional Assays*

Proliferation Assay

Peripheral blood leukocytes (PBL) were resuspended in medium consisting of RPMI 1640, 2 m*M* glutamine, 100 U/ml penicillin, 100 μg/ml streptomycin, and 20% heat-inactivated fetal calf serum or autologous plasma (complete medium).

PBL (10^5/well) were cultured in triplicate in 96-well flat-bottomed microculture plates (Costar) in a total volume of 0.2 ml. Cell cultures were stimulated with three different concentrations of phytohemagglutinin (PHA)-A (0.5, 1, and 5 μg/ml) and with a combination of PHA/PMA (PHA 0.5 μg/ml and PMA 1 ng/ml). Cell cultures were incubated at 37 °C for 72 h in a humidified atmosphere containing 5% CO_2 in air. Proliferation was assessed by adding [^{3}H]-thymidine (1 μCi/well) during the last 18 h of the cell culture.

Cytokine Assay

One-milliliter aliquots of cell suspension containing 2×10^6 viable PBL were distributed in 24-well microplates and stimulated by adding 1 ml of complete medium containing PHA at a final concentration of 0.5 μg/ml, or PHA plus PMA (PMA final concentration 1 ng/ml). Nonstimulated control PBL were prepared in parallel. Two replicates were prepared for subject and treatment. Cultures were incubated at 37 °C in a humidified atmosphere of CO_2 and 95% air.

Analysis of IL-2 mRNA Expression

After 72 h of stimulation with PHA or PHA plus PMA, PBLs were collected and washed with ice-cold PBS (pH 7.4). Cells were lysed in denaturation buffer and total RNA was extracted using the Stratagene RNA isolation kit. RNA concentrations were adjusted to 1 μg/μl. Reverse transcriptase (RTP) was performed with oligo $d(T)_{16}$ priming (60 min at 37 °C, 10 min at 95 °C).

Polymerase chain reaction (PRC) was conducted following the manufacturer's instructions (Gene Amp Kit, Perkin Elmer). Thus, 2 μl sample cDNA and 2 μl BD1 (internal standard for IL-2) were used as templates. Amplification of IL-2 transcripts was performed as follows: 45 s at 94 °C, 1 min at 60 °C, 1.5 min at 72 °C, 30 cycles; 45 s at 94 °C, 1 min at 60 °C, 7 min at 72 °C, one cycle. For each PCR a serial dilution of BD1 (10 to 10^{-5} amol) was co-amplified to establish a standard curve for IL-2-specific transcripts. PCR products were analyzed on a 2% agarose gel containing ethidium bromide.

For the dot-blot analysis, the PCR products of the samples and standard curve (BD1) were diluted 1:10 in TE buffer (pH 8.0), loaded in duplicates on nitrocellulose (Genescreen, NEN Dupont), and fixed under UV radiation.

Hybridization was performed under standard conditions with a specific 33P–IL-2 antisense probe which was end-labeled by T4 kinase (Stratagene) before use. The nitrocellulose was exposed to an X-ray film (in the presence of Strategene reference). Spots were cut from the nitrocellulose and radioactivity was determined by liquid scintillation counting.

Statistics

Statistics were performed using the Number Cruncher Statistical Systems software (NCSS, Kaysville, Utah 84037). The influence of single independent factors was assessed by classic one-way analysis of variance (ANOVA). When the assumption of normality was not valid, the Kruskal-Wallis one-way ANOVA on ranks was used as a nonparametric alternative.

Results

Peripheral Blood Lymphocyte Subsets

Total lymphocyte counts showed a trend of lower values in the group at risk of malnutrition compared with the well-nourished group, while the malnourished group had lower values when compared with the group at risk of malnutrition (Fig. 1a). However, this trend did not reach statistical significance. No real lymphopenia was observed in any of the groups. No differences were observed for CD3+ lymphocytes (total T cells; Fig. 1b), or for CD4+ or CD45RA/RO CD4+ T cell subsets (data not shown). B cell (CD19+) counts were similar for the three MNA categories and fell within the normal range (data not shown). CD8+ T cells followed a similar pattern to total lymphocytes and were lower in the malnourished group. Again, statistical significance was not reached (Fig. 1c).

A lymphocyte subpopulation like natural killer (NK) cells, which is in part CD3–, was not specifically characterized in the present study. One could speculate that this particular subset is reduced in the malnourished group and could contribute to the changes observed in the total lymphocyte counts. However, no abnormal values in the other leukocyte populations were observed.

The red blood cell compartment showed a significant difference between the well-nourished and malnourished groups ($p < 0.05$ ANOVA and Kruskal-Wallis one-way ANOVA on ranks tests), as shown by the hemoglobin and hematocrit levels (Fig. 2). When the lymphocyte subpopulations were compared between the anemic and nonanemic groups, fewer CD8+ cells were observed in the former (Fig. 3).

When groups were defined on the basis of serum albumin concentrations (group 1 <35 g/l, group 2 between 35 and 40 g/l, and group 3 >40 g/l) the differences in total lymphocyte counts and in the different lymphocyte subsets were still more subtle than for the MNA categories (data not shown).

In conclusion, in this trial we could not show an association between nutritional status – as defined by MNA, albumin, or anemia – and lymphocyte counts. Only a subtle change was observed for total lymphocytes and for CD8+ cells. As mentioned above, it is possible that a specific lymphocyte subset, such as NK, is more sensitive to nutritional status but this was not determined in the present study.

Serum Immunoglobulins

No differences were observed for serum IgG and IgM concentrations among the three MNA categories. In contrast, a higher concentration of serum IgA (Fig. 4) was detected in the malnourished group ($p < 0.05$ by ANOVA and Krus-

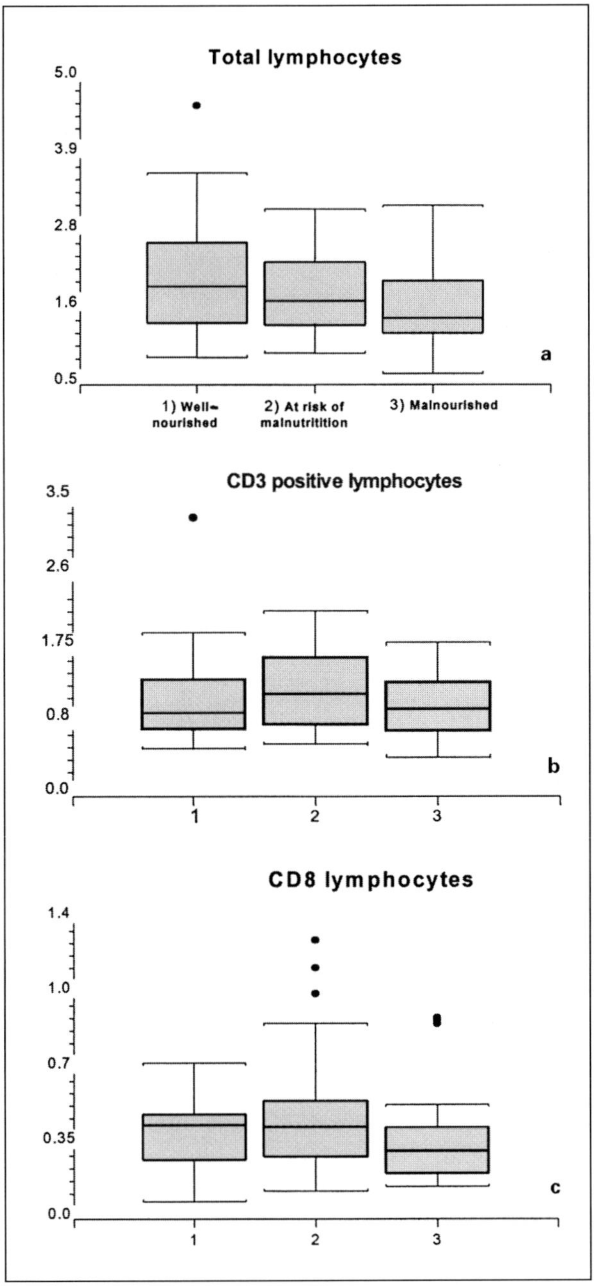

Fig. 1. Total lymphocyte counts (10^3/ml) were higher in group 1 but the difference did not reach statistical significance (**a**); a similar pattern was observed for CD8+ cells (**c**), whereas similar counts for CD3+ cells were found in all three groups (**b**).

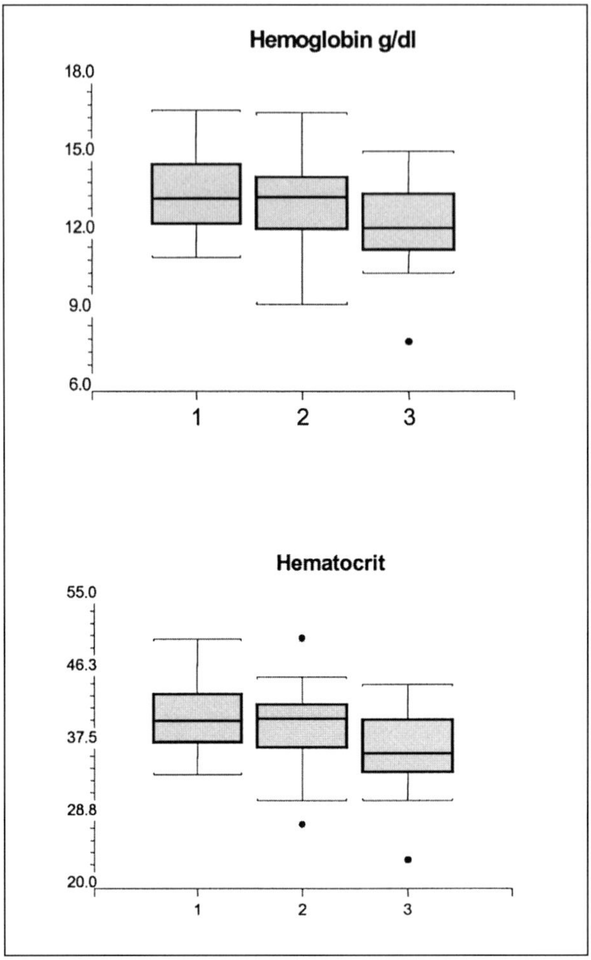

Fig. 2. Hemoglobin (g/dl) and hematocrit (%) in the three MNA categories. Significant differences for hemoglobin ($p = 0.02$) and hematocrit ($p = 0.018$) were observed between the well-nourished and malnourished groups according to the Kruskal-Wallis one-way ANOVA on ranks test.

kal-Wallis one-way ANOVA on ranks) when compared with the group at risk of malnutrition.

When patients were divided into anemic and nonanemic groups, a nonsignificant trend showing higher IgA concentrations in the anemic group was also observed (data not shown). In contrast, no difference in immunoglobulin levels for any of the isotypes was observed when groups were defined according to albumin concentrations.

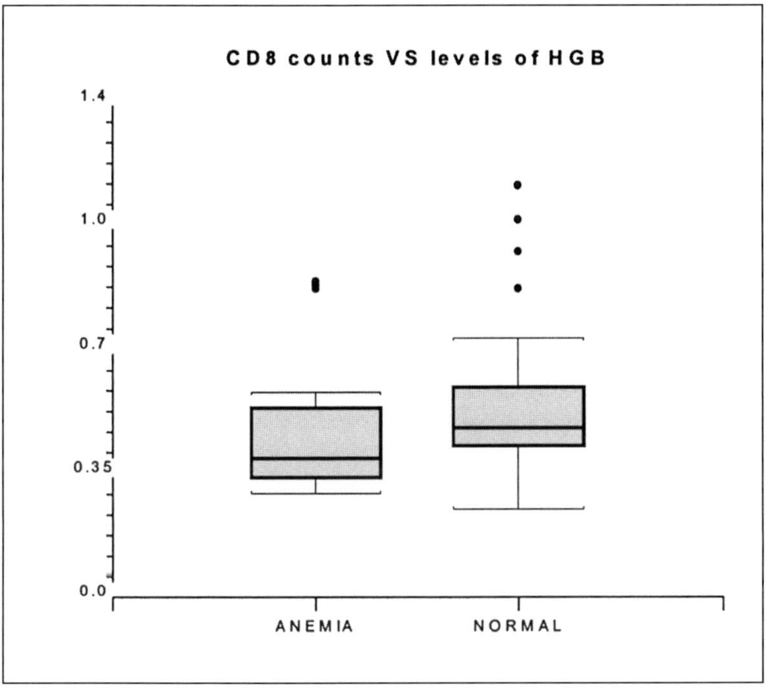

3

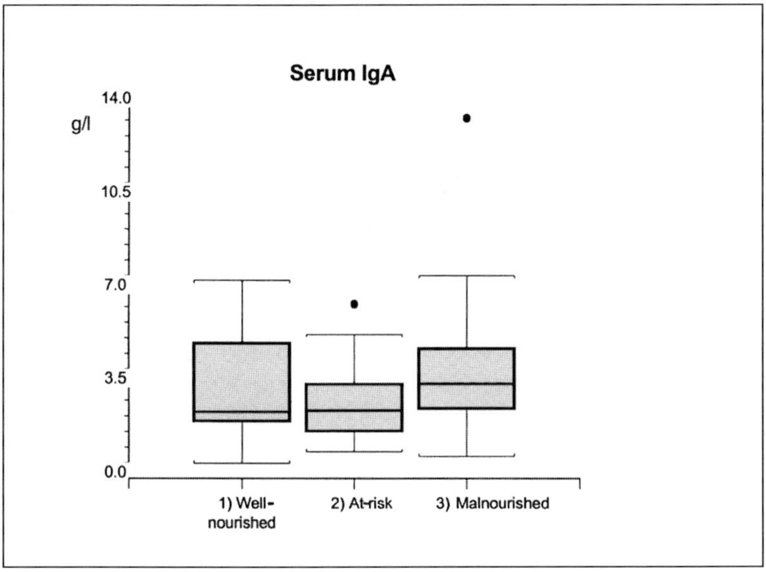

4

Fig. 3. Lymphocyte counts ($\times 10^3$): $p = 0.07$ between groups.
Fig. 4. Comparison of serum IgA concentrations; $p < 0.05$ between malnourished and at-risk groups by Kruskal-Wallis one-way ANOVA on ranks test.

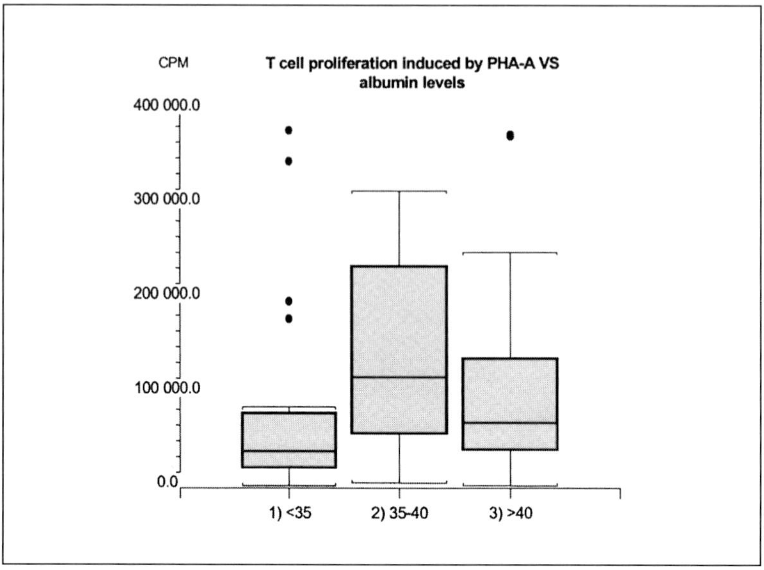

Fig. 5. T cell proliferation (CPM) after 72 h stimulation with PHA-A 0.5 µg/ml ($p < 0.05$ between groups 1 and 2).

Proliferation and Activation of Mitogen-Treated PBL

A clear stimulation of T cell proliferation was achieved with PHA, at all doses tested, and with PHA/PMA combined treatments. However, [^{3}H]-thymidine incorporation was similar for the three categories defined by the MNA score in all conditions tested (data not shown). In agreement with the proliferative activity, no differences in CD25 expression (marker of activation) on CD3+ T cells were observed comparing the different MNA groups 72 h after *in vitro* stimulation.

When groups were defined according to albumin levels, [^{3}H]-thymidine incorporation was lower (Fig. 5) in the group with a plasma albumin of <35 g/l ($p <$ 0.05 by Kruskal-Wallis one-way ANOVA on ranks).

IL-2-Specific mRNA

IL-2-specific mRNA was determined by a semiquantitative method combining RT-PCR and a dot-blot technique. IL-2 transcription was low to undetectable in nonstimulated control cells and PHA-treated PBL. In contrast, IL-2-specific mRNA expression in PBL was clearly higher, compared with the controls, after the combined treatment using PHA/PMA. Higher quantities of specific IL-2 mRNA were detected in the MNA "well-nourished" category compared with the other categories. Although this difference did not reach statistical significance ($p = 0.06$), it shows an obvious trend (Fig. 6).

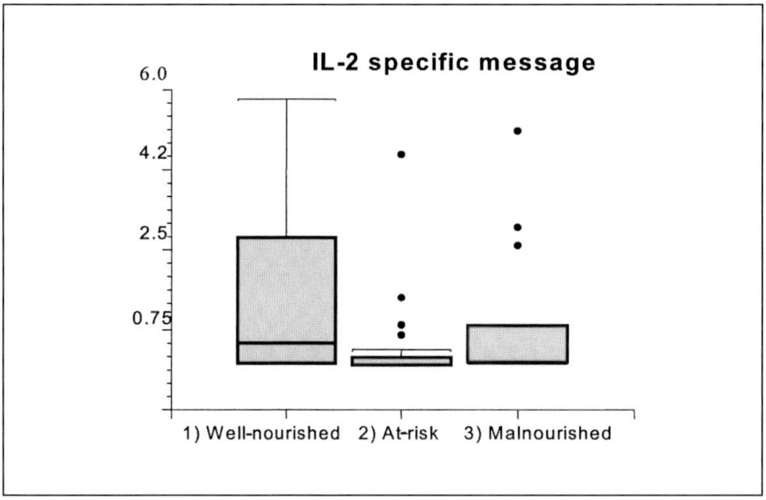

Fig. 6. Attomoles of mRNA specific for IL-2 ($\times 10^2$); $p = 0.06$, group 1 *vs.* groups 2 and 3 (Kruskal-Wallis one-way ANOVA on ranks test).

Discussion

The aim of our study was to establish a correlation between a clinical tool, such as the MNA, for screening for malnutrition in the elderly, and some biological immune markers. This appeared to be of major interest since impaired immune function in the elderly population often leads to a fatal outcome. We and others have hypothesized that a part of the immune deficit observed in elderly people is caused by nutritional deficiencies and not exclusively by an aging genetic program [8, 9]. In the past it has also been shown that malnutrition is a common subclinical underlying condition in this population [5].

In this study we explored two major sets of indices reflecting the cellular basis of immune dysfunction and its potential association with malnutrition. The first included the determination of serum levels of different antibody isotypes and blood lymphocyte populations; the second was related to the capacity of immune cells to react *in vitro* to activation signals such as polyclonal mitogens. IL-2 induction is closely related to lymphocyte proliferation and reflects the capacity of T lymphocytes to enter cell cycle upon (antigen) mitogen stimulation. This is a basic and crucial event in any specific immune response.

In this study good proliferation activity was observed for the three doses of PHA tested and also for the combination of PHA/PMA. No clear differences or dose-response type of pattern were observed among the different treatments (data not shown). However, IL-2-specific mRNA was only clearly upregulated by the combined PHA/PMA stimulus, while no clear specific message induction was observed above the resting levels with single PHA treatment at whatever dose tested.

Comparing the levels of IL-2 mRNA expression after 72 h of PHA/PMA stimulation among different MNA categories revealed a higher level of IL-2 transcripts in the well-nourished group (Fig. 6). This may suggest that the diminished IL-2 production previously reported in the elderly [2] could in part be linked to nutritional status. In addition, since PMA interacts directly with protein kinase C (PKC), a defect in T cell activation in the elderly may rather be associated with an altered expression of receptors (receptor densities) or with the physical status of plasma membrane than with the distal events in the genetic activation by antigens.

In this study, our failure to detect a clear induction of IL-2 mRNA with a single PHA treatment was probably related to the late mRNA sampling rather than to an impairment in signal transduction. The high proliferative stimulation seems to suggest this interpretation.

Concerning the lymphocyte populations, total lymphocyte counts were within the normal range for all the groups and lymphopenia was not detectable. Nevertheless, in both the malnourished group (according to the MNA category) and the anemic group, total lymphocyte and CD8+ T cell numbers were lower than in the other groups. However, this diminution was not statistically significant.

There is some discrepancy in the effect of age and malnutrition on the NK populations. Unfortunately this subset of lymphocytes could not be determined in this study. In contrast, lymphopenia has previously been described in elderly people and was associated with low CD4+ counts [10]. It is a matter of debate, though, whether low CD4+ T cell counts are related to malnutrition or to a chronic inflammatory condition [11].

Conclusion

In conclusion, although the population of elderly people included in this study showed markers of malnutrition, the deficiencies were not severe enough to alter the homeostasis of the immune system. In fact, MNA detection of malnutrition seems to anticipate other biochemical markers of malnutrition and indicates a population at risk, before the physiology of the immune response is profoundly altered.

References

1. Thoman ML, Weigle WO. The cellular bases of immunosenescence. *Adv Immunol* 1989; 46: 221–61.
2. Nagel JE, Chopra RK, Chrest FJ, *et al.* Decreased proliferation, interleukin-2 synthesis, and interleukin-2 receptor expression are accompanied by decreased mRNA expression in phytohemagglutinin-stimulated cells from elderly donors. *J Clin Invest* 1988; 81: 1096–102.

3. Proust JJ, Filburn CR, Harrison SA, Buchholz MA, Nordin AA. Age related defect in signal transduction during lectin activation of murine lymphocytes. *J Immunol* 1987; 139: 1472–8.
4. Franceschi C, Monti D, Sansoni P, Cossarizza A. The immunology of exceptional individuals: the lesson of centenarians. *Immunol Today* 1995; 16: 12–6.
5. Guigoz Y, Vellas B, Garry PJ. Assesing the nutritional status of the elderly: the Mini Nutritional Assessment as part of the geriatric evaluation. *Nutr Rev* 1996; 54: S59–65.
6. Euronut SENECA Investigators. Nutritional status: haematology and albumin. *Eur J Clin Nutr* 1991; 45 (suppl 3): 43–52.
7. WHO. *Nutritional anemias;* technical report series, No 405. Geneva: World Health Organisation, 1968.
8. Chandra RK. Effect of vitamin and trace-element supplementation on immune responses and infection in elderly subjects. *Lancet* 1992; 340: 1124–7.
9. Chandra RK. Nutritional regulation of immunity and risk of infection in old age. *Immunology* 1989; 67: 141–7.
10. Rae IM, Alexander HD, Crockard AD, Morris TCM. CD4 lymphopenia in very old people. *Lancet* 1996; 347: 328–9.
11. Belmin J, Ortega MN, Bruhat A, Mercadier A, Valensi P. CD4 lymphopenia in elderly patients. *Lancet* 1996; 347: 911.

Discussion

Dr. Steenhout: Dr. Schiffrin, your data on IgA are very interesting. We have recently conducted a study in infants with criteria of malnutrition, and we also found an increase of IgA in saliva. I would be interested in your opinion on the mechanism. It is a good thing to identify indicators, but we also need to know the underlying pathophysiology. Is it related to infectious disease perhaps? Have you found that patients with low MNA scores have a higher frequency of infectious disease? I'm concerned that the trials may have included patients with different pathologies, which could affect the indices that were measured.

Dr. Schiffrin: I think we can assume that the IgA isotype comes mainly from GALT (gut-associated lymphoid tissue). We know that elderly people have increased gut permeability – the mucosal barrier works less efficiently and there is a greater antigen and infection challenge. This is speculation, but the mucosal barrier is probably more altered in patients with a low MNA score and a low hemoglobin. We know that anemic patients have reduced gut perfusion and increased permeability, so there is increased passage of antigens and a greater IgA response. I think we can assume that the inefficient mucosal barrier allows more macromolecules to pass, leading to a greater IgA response.

Dr. Vellas: I have two comments. First, I believe it is important that we identify the extent to which MNA is a marker of nutrition and the extent to which it is a marker of frailty. This could be important for the future. Second, in relation to MNA and immunological function, it seemed in the study we did in Toulouse that the people with low MNA scores had malnutrition, because they had a decreased energy intake. However, they had no inflammation and no evidence of other disease. I think impairment of immune function is most likely to be a result of hypercatabolism and of malnutrition plus disease, but not of malnutrition alone. This may be an important point.

Dr. Schiffrin: I agree with you. We were looking specifically for inflammatory markers and evidence of a catabolic state which would result in a modification of the immune response. The Toulouse population was too healthy to resolve this issue!

Dr. Vellas: One of our exclusion criteria was acute disease.

Dr. Morley: Most immune functions show a subtle decrease with age. Malnutrition on the whole makes that worse, particularly if severe. The only immune function that I'm aware of that does not decline with age but does decline with malnutrition is the CD4 count. We have shown this in an older age group and it was also shown many years ago in a pediatric population [1]. You did not present CD4 data. Do you have such data?

Dr. Schiffrin: CD4 didn't change or showed only a proportional increase because CD8 and NK cells decreased.

Dr. Morley: That suggests that your population had minimal malnutrition.

Dr. Camilla: I have two questions. First, how old does one need to be to be called elderly? I've seen data from 55 to over 75! Second, MNA looks like any other kind of global assessment of nutritional risk. How good is it for interventional studies? Don't we need to correlate the scores with functional variables other than fancy immunological tests?

Dr. Guesry: I'm not going to tell you how old you should be to be called elderly, but MNA has been validated in a certain age range, and outside that range it has not been validated. So for your first question the answer is in Yves Guigoz' article!

Dr. Guigoz: Regarding interventions, we have already used MNA assessment during an intervention study [see Arnaud-Battandier *et al.*, this volume]; we now need more intervention studies, which is the next step.

Reference

1. Kaiser FE, Morley JE. Idiopathic CD4+ T lymphopenia in orlder persons. *J Am Geriatr Soc* 1994; 42 (12): 1291–4.

Mini Nutritional Assessment (MNA): Research and Practice in the Elderly:
B. Vellas; P.J. Garry; Y. Guigoz (eds),
Nestlé Nutrition Workshop Series Clinical & Performance Programme, Vol. 1, pp. 35–40,
Nestec Ltd.; Vevey/S. Karger AG, Basel, © 1999.

Comparative Nutrition Evaluation with the Mini Nutritional Assessment and the Nutritional Risk Assessment Scale

P. Oster, B.M. Rost, U. Velte and G. Schlierf

Geriatrisches Zentrum Bethanien, Klinikum der Universität, Heidelberg, Germany

Malnutrition in geriatric hospital inpatients over 75 years old is one of the strongest indicators of a poor outcome, including mortality. A subjective rating of the nutritional status correlated strongly ($p < 0.001$) with the subsequent mortality at follow-up times of 6, 18, and 30 months after discharge from hospital. Mortality was twice as high in malnourished patients as in normally nourished patients and four times higher than in overweight patients [1]. We therefore developed an assessment of nutritional risk in order to identify possible nutritional interventions; this also included risk indicators for the future development of malnutrition owing to factors that might be related to the hospital admission itself [2]. In the present study we compared our nutritional assessment – the nutritional risk assessment scale (NuRAS) – with the Mini Nutritional Assessment (MNA) [3].

Patients and Methods

All patients, admitted consecutively to one acute geriatric and one rehabilitation ward, were eligible for the study; both assessments were performed by one interviewer during the first three days after admission. Drug treatments and body weight were taken from the patients' records, and height was calculated from the knee-heel distance.

The MNA was performed after Guigoz *et al.* [3], and the NuRAS as described by Nikolaus *et al.* [2] (Table 1). In the MNA, points are given for positive nutrition factors, resulting in a high score for good nutritional status (24 points or more), an intermediate risk zone (17–23.5 points), and a low score < 17 indicating malnutrition. The NuRAS assessment simply identifies single risk factors that

Table 1. Yes/no questions of the Nutritional Risk Assessment Scale [2]

1.	Has the patient a gastrointestinal disorder?
2.	Has the patient a chronic disease with pain?
3.	Has the patient swallowing problems?
4.	Has the patient difficulty in cutting food?
5.	Has the patient a gait disorder?
6.	Does the patient report an unexpected weight loss (>5 kg during the last 6 months)?
7.	Does the patient complain of poor appetite or change in appetite?
8.	Does the patient show poor oral health or chewing problems?
9.	Is the patient taking five or more prescription drugs and/or has a high consumption of alcohol (>3 drinks/day for a man, 1 drink/day for a woman) or of cigarettes (>10 cigarettes/day)?
10.	Does the patient show clinical evidence of mental/cognitive impairment?
11.	Does the patient show clinical evidence of depressive illness?
12.	Does the patient suffer from social isolation?

could result in nutritional interventions. For example, problems with teeth, swallowing, digestion, or loss of weight are analyzed separately, while in the MNA they are summarized under "anorexia."

Results

Of 55 potential subjects, 50 could be included in the study (two refused, in one the anthropometric data could not be obtained, and two were not able to answer the questions because of aphasia). The average age of the participants was 78.4 years (range 59–95), 34 were female and 16 male, 34 were from the acute geriatric ward and 16 from the rehabilitation ward. Their average height was 159.5 cm (range 132–183) and their weight 65.3 kg (38.9–105.2), resulting in a mean body mass index of 26.5 kg/m^2 (13.9–41.6).

The risk scores in the two assessments correlated highly ($p < 0.01$), especially in the upper (normal) and lower (malnutrition) range of the MNA; variability was greatest in the intermediate risk zone of the MNA in comparison with the NuRAS risk factors (Fig. 1). If the simple subjective judgment of the physician was plotted against the MNA total score (Fig. 2), all patients classified as cachectic scored <17 points on the MNA and the majority of patients subjectively rated as undernourished scored <17 points, only three were in the risk zone, and none scored in the normal zone.

The time required for the performance of the assessments was highly variable. The MNA tended to be more time-consuming (about double the time), mainly because of the anthropometric measurements. In NuRAS, the question relating to the social situation needed a lot of time to answer for some patients. The NuRAS can be performed in 5–10 min.

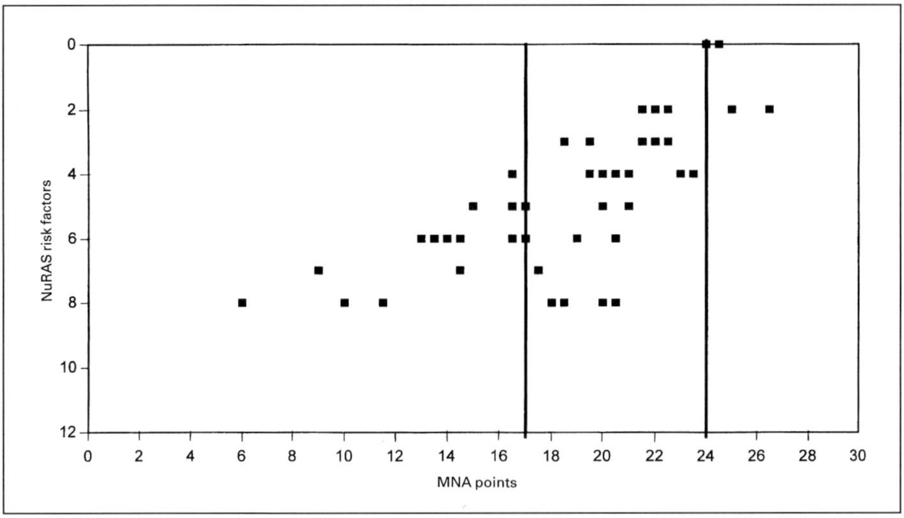

Fig. 1. Risk factors NuRAS against points in the MNA; vertical bars mark the risk zone of the MNA.

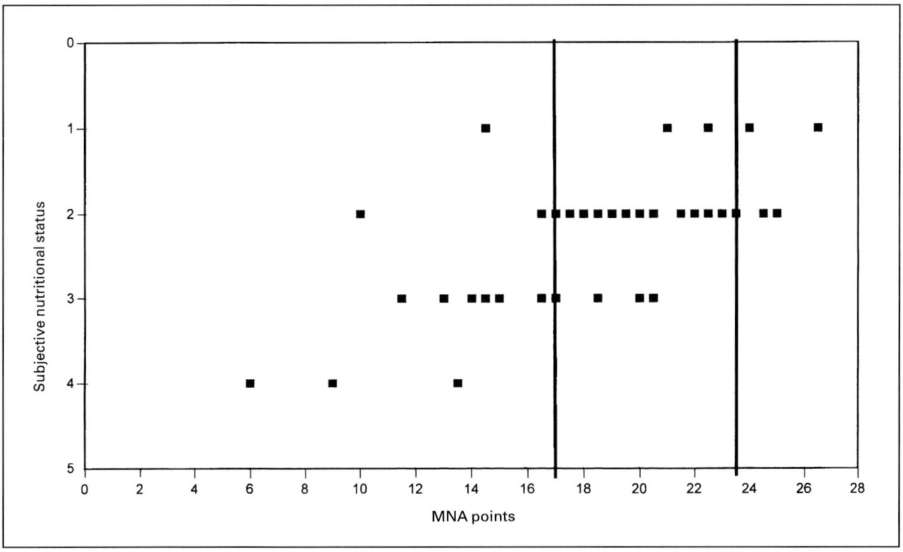

Fig. 2. MNA points plotted against subjective classification of nutritional status in (1) obese, (2) normal, (3) undernourished, and (4) cachectic patients.

From the MNA scores there was a total of 31 possible nutrition interventions, and from the NuRAS, 26; this amounted overall to 548 nutritional interventions resulting from the MNA and 434 resulting from the NuRAS.

Discussion

In geriatric medicine, malnutrition is a strong indicator of poor outcome, including increased mortality, for many diseases. In institutionalized elderly patients, it is one of the most prevalent health problems [1, 4, 5]. Therefore every effort must be made to diagnose undernutrition. In this study we showed that a simple clinical assessment of nutritional status by the physician, classifying the patient as cachectic, undernourished, normally nourished, or overnourished, can be as good as a battery of biochemical and anthropometric tests [6]. Despite the ease of the diagnosis, malnutrition is still one of the most neglected problems in geriatric medicine. Because of this, formal assessment procedures like the MNA and the NuRAS have been developed, which are able to combine a nutritional diagnosis with suggestions for possible nutritional intervention. The time required to do these tests can be as short as 5 min, especially when incorporated in a comprehensive geriatric assessment.

In our study, 548 possible nutritional interventions could be identified in 50 patients as a result of the MNA assessment, and 434 as a result of the NuRAS. The difference is mainly explained by the section of the MNA dealing with specific food items and fluid intake. In the NuRAS the questions about the social situation and chronic pain are helpful in identifying possible nutritional interventions. A formal nutritional assessment is an educational tool for physicians (and other health workers) in training, while the somewhat complicated anthropometric measurements may well please the patient. Sometimes, however, anthropometry is impossible or unreliable (for example, when there is edema) or may produce unnecessary difficulties (as with an amputation).

Every procedure must be as simple as possible, especially when performed in young elderly and generally healthy populations, where only a few positive results can be expected. A screening procedure or an abbreviated MNA [Rubenstein LZ, this volume] should suffice; in the typical geriatric patient, where a formal comprehensive geriatric assessment is indicated, a nutritional assessment such as the MNA or the NuRAS should be incorporated. The questions and their interpretation must be as clear as possible, for example they should be outlined in an instruction manual (see question "living alone" in the MNA, because living alone can be either a good sign or a risk factor). Finally, the interventions resulting from the assessment should be effective and should ideally be followed by improved scores in the nutrition assessment, as could be shown by Battandier *et al.* [this volume] with the MNA, leading to a better quality of life for the geriatric patient.

References

1. Rampmeier J. *Einfluss von vierteljährlichen rehabilitativen Hausbesuchen bei hochbetagten geriatrischen Patienten nach der Krankenhausentlassung auf nachfolgende Krankenhausaufenthalte und Mortalität.* Heidelberg: University of Heidelberg, 1996 (Dissertation).
2. Nikolaus T, Bach M, Siezen S, Volkert D, Oster P, Schlierf G. Assessment of nutritional risk in the elderly. *Ann Nutr Metab* 1995; 39: 340–5.
3. Guigoz Y, Vellas B, Garry P. Assessing the nutritional status of the elderly: the Mini Nutritional Assessment as part of the geriatric evaluation. *Nutr Rev* 1996; 54(II): S59–65.
4. Seiler W, Stähelin H. Besondere Aspekte der Malnutrition in der Geriatrie. *Schweiz Med Wochenschr* 1995; 125: 149–58.
5. Volkert D. *Ernährung im Alter.* Wiesbaden: Quelle und Meyer, 1997.
6. Volkert D, Kruse W, Oster P, Schlierf G. Malnutrition in geriatric patients: diagnostic and prognostic significance of nutritional parameters. *Ann Nutr Metab* 1992; 36: 97–112.

Discussion

Dr. Ferry: A question for Dr. Oster about the item "living alone" in the MNA: does this mean "being isolated" or "being able to live alone," that is, not in a nursing home. There is a big difference between the two.

Dr. Oster: You get a point in the MNA for living alone. This might be good, but it might be very bad if you are isolated and depressive.

Dr. Cohendy: I do not agree that the first block of the MNA questionnaire is difficult to calculate. We have calculated more than 400 questionnaires, and found no special difficulty. Perhaps this is because our aims were somewhat different. For us, the aim was to assess risk; for Dr. Oster it was to describe the mechanism leading to malnutrition in elderly patients. In my view, it would be desirable if at the end of this conference we could say whether the MNA is a tool for assessing risk of malnutrition or for assessing the mechanism leading to malnutrition.

Dr. Oster: I was quoting the opinions of my coworkers, who really performed the assessment. Knowing that subjective assessment is also quite reliable, they suggested that it might be sufficient just to have the subjective rating of a physician or a nutritionist. Rather than stopping doing the MNA because it is too complicated, it would be preferable to get a subjective idea of whether malnutrition is present or not.

Dr. Vellas: I'd like to remind you that the MNA was designed to be used in the clinic. If patients go to see a physician because of anorexia or weight loss, the clinician needs to examine them as well as taking a history. Anthropometric measurements are really useful clinical markers in this regard. It would be hard for the physician to ask for $ 50 if they don't touch the patient! Also, when anyone learns to use the MNA, with all its questions, they are learning how to do a nutritional assessment. The MNA was designed for clinic-based nutritional assessment, not as a fast screening tool for public health.

Dr. Arnaud-Battandier: We observed in France that some general practitioners in private practice consider the anthropometry difficult to do and time-consuming. So we proposed that they not do this block in certain circumstances. When using MNA for diagnostic purposes, even if you have the maximum value for anthropometry, the score will still be below 17 if the other indicators are negative. Of course, to follow the patient with MNA, you need anthropometric measurements.

Dr. Shimmler: I think this touches on the issue of the use of MNA: is it to assess status or to measure risk? What you are saying is that if you want to get a measure of nutritional status at a particular point in time, and if the score is going to be below 17 whatever the body measurements, then you've answered the question already: their nutritional status is low.

But if you want to predict the future outcome and risk, then you will need the additional part to complete the assessment.

Dr. Salvá: If you want to do a nutritional assessment, you need to measure body mass index or some other anthropometric index. It is very important to know if there has been weight loss, and how much change there has been. When we do the MNA, it is not enough to look at the total MNA score; we need to look at each of the questions, because if there is a diagnosis of malnutrition, we need to plan an intervention program. Only by obtaining anthropometric measures can we follow the patient's progress.

Dr. Morley: Your point is very well taken. Dr. Miller and I have done two studies, one at UCLA and one in St. Louis, looking at the ability of residents to recognize malnutrition [1]. If you ask someone "Does this person look malnourished?", they can often give you the right answer, but they are incapable of seeing it unless you ask the question. That is where I think anthropometry becomes very important; it trains people to understand and to look for malnutrition. I would strongly encourage maintaining the anthropometric score component.

Dr. Chumlea: I have a comment about MNA as an instrument for multicultural use. There may be problems with asking questions in the right way. For example, Japanese or Chinese people may have a different perception from Westerners about what constitutes fruits and vegetables. That needs to be looked into if you're planning to use the MNA in other cultures.

Reference

1. Miller DK, Morley JE, Rubenstein LZ, Pietruszka FM, Strome LS. Formal geriatric assessment instruments and the care of the older general medical outpatients. *J Am Geriatr Soc* 1990; 38 (6): 645–51.

Mini Nutritional Assessment (MNA): Research and Practice in the Elderly:
B. Vellas; P.J. Garry; Y. Guigoz (eds),
Nestlé Nutrition Workshop Series Clinical & Performance Programme, Vol. 1, pp. 41–60,
Nestec Ltd.; Vevey/S. Karger AG, Basel, © 1999.

MNA and Odor Perception

Martijn I. Griep, Tony F. Mets, Kris Collys, Dominique Verté, Gino Verleye, Ingrid Ponjaert-Kristoffersen and Desire L. Massart

VUB Free University of Brussels, Faculty of Medicine and Pharmacy; STATAP bvba, Ghent, Belgium

Part 1

Malnutrition, General Health, Body Composition, Dental State, and Odor Perception

Many studies show that odor perception declines with age, while diminished odor perception is associated with poor general health and various diseases [1–3]. Though it has been suggested that many nutrients play a role in odor perception, and elderly people are prone to develop undetected malnutrition [4–8], results from previous published studies on the relation between odor perception and nutrition are conflicting [9–12]. It has been suggested that in elderly people living independently at home without obvious nutritional deficiencies, health problems are more important in explaining diminished odor perception than nutritional state, as measured by anthropometry. Muscle tissue diminishes with age owing to reduced mobility and a sedentary lifestyle; in combination with poor general health, this might cause diminished odor perception. Early detection of diminished odor perception might therefore be an indication of physical deterioration [13]. On the other hand, it has been suggested that declining odor perception can cause changes in food consumption and diminished food appreciation [14], as illustrated in Figure 1. The sensory properties of food (for example, flavor, texture) are important determinants of food consumption [15]. Ninety percent of food flavors consist of volatile odors [16], and changes in palatability or sensory quality of food can mainly be ascribed to a declining perception of odors [15].

Poor oral health is widespread among the elderly. Caries, periodontal disease, defective or ill-fitting dentures, and poor oral or denture hygiene are common [17, 18]. In addition, missing teeth can have detrimental effects on mastication, oral

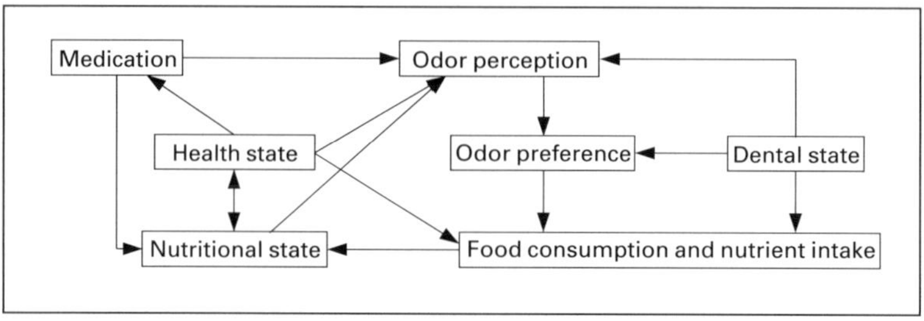

Fig. 1. Overview of age-related phenomena under investigation.

health, and nutrition [19]. It has been suggested that the proportion of persons with an insufficient intake of nutrients is higher among edentulous individuals than in dentate persons [20]. Moreover, the oral cavity is an area where micro-organisms may metabolize a variety of substances to produce malodors. Such malodors may cause a masking or adaptation of the olfactory receptors, hence leading to diminished food odor perception [21].

With increasing age, the combined influence of odor perception and oral health on nutritional state is to be expected, since both odor perception and dental health may affect food consumption [22].

It has been well established that nutritional and oral problems are widespread among elderly people living in retirement homes, where from a functional point of view both the degree of dependency and general health are expected to influence nutritional status. We therefore explored which age-associated factors – such as poor oral health, degree of dependency, body composition, diminished odor perception, and diminished functionality – are accompanied by an increased risk of malnutrition. In Figure 1, the different age-related phenomena under investigation are shown.

In the first experiment, using a validated screening tool for the detection of malnutrition – the Mini Nutritional Assessment (MNA) – elderly people living independently at home in the community were studied. In the second experiment, elderly people living in retirement homes with varying degrees of dependency were included.

Subjects and Methods

Odor Perception

To determine odor perception, the detection threshold for isoamylacetate (fruity banana/pear odor) was determined as the lowest detectable odor concentration. The described method has been widely used with many substances and has been calibrated in previous studies [23–25]. The isoamylacetate solutions were prepared according to the procedure and substances described by Laska & Hudson [26]. Odors were presented in 250 ml polyethylene squeeze bottles containing 40 ml of solution and equipped with a flip-up spout with an interchangeable nose piece made of Teflon. Each person received a series of paired bottles (one blank containing the solvent only and one containing the odor). According to the so-called "forced choice" paradigm, the participants were asked to sniff and to indicate which one smelled stronger. An inter-trial interval of 30 s was chosen to allow recovery from adaptation. Detection thresholds were determined by using an ascending method of limits, starting at the lowest of the 14 prepared concentrations. Threshold was reached when five subsequent pairs were correctly indicated.

All measurements were carried out in a well-ventilated and quiet room. Gas chromatography verification showed that headspace concentrations of freshly prepared solutions in the bottles remained constant over the whole testing period. During preliminary testing with this procedure, in which odor thresholds were obtained from 25 healthy young persons (aged 19–25 years, mean 22.3), it was shown that the mean threshold fell within the range found by others [27].

Dental State

Concomitant with the sensory tests, oral examinations were carried out in a standardized way by a dentist (K.C.). The number of natural teeth and dentures was counted and type of dentures was identified.

Mini Nutritional Assessment

The MNA is a rapid assessment tool and was used to evaluate the risk of malnutrition [28]. The protocol comprises 18 items involving anthropometry, general assessments, dietary assessments, and subjective assessment. MNA has recently been validated and can accurately assess nutritional status of elderly people as normal or well-nourished, borderline or at risk of malnutrition, and frankly malnourished. The scoring categorizes each person as well-nourished (≥ 24 points), at risk of malnutrition (17–24 points), and malnourished (<17 points).

General Health and Body Composition

The general health status was determined by the Medical Outcome Study (MOS) scores. The scale has been validated by Stewart *et al.* [29]. The MOS scale allows a quantitative measure of functional health of elderly people, based on the following concepts:

Physical functioning – the extent to which health interferes with a number of daily activities such as sporting, walking, shopping.

Role functioning – the extent to which health interferes with working or household activities.

Social functioning – the extent to which health interferes with social activities such as visiting friends and family.

Mental functioning – general mood, well-being, depression, and fear.
Perceived health – general judgement concerning current state of health.
Perceived pain – amount of pain experienced.

The items were chosen to represent six health concepts, using the WHO definition of health [29].

Anthropometric measures were obtained to assess physical deterioration and the distribution of fat and muscle. The variables chosen were those used in similar studies of nutritional status [30] and odor perception [31]: mid-arm circumference (MAC), triceps skinfold thickness (TSF), mid-calf circumference (MCC), abdominal circumference (measured at the level of the umbilicus), and hip circumference (at the maximum protuberance of the buttocks). All persons were weighed in kilograms, and height was measured in meters. Circumferences were measured in millimeters using a flexible tape measure, and skinfold thicknesses in millimeters by a calibrated caliper. Muscle circumferences and areas were calculated as general indicators of protein status, muscle atrophy or protein-energy malnutrition. Arm muscle circumference (AMC) was derived as:

$$\text{AMC} = \text{MAC} - (\pi \cdot \text{TSF}).$$

Arm muscle area (AMA), corrected for bone (AMAB), was derived as:

$$\text{AMAB} = [(\text{MAC} - \pi \cdot \text{TSF})^2/(4 \cdot \pi)] - 10 \text{ (men)},$$

or

$$[(\text{MAC} - \pi \cdot \text{TSF})^2/(4 \cdot \pi)] - 6.5 \text{ (women)}.$$

For measuring the amount of body fat, different measures of subcutaneous fat were calculated. Body mass index (BMI) was derived from weight and height as a global measure of body fatness. As measures of subcutaneous fat, upper arm subcutaneous fat area was calculated as:

$$[\text{MAC} \cdot \text{TSF}/2] - [\pi \cdot (\text{TSF})^2/4].$$

Drugs

Since odor perception was expected to be associated with both nutritional state and use of drugs, the following procedure was used to partition the persons into three groups: those taking no drugs; those taking drugs expected to influence odor perception; and those taking other types of drugs. Based on published studies by others, we identified active compounds in drugs which would be expected to have effects on odor perception [2, 32, 33]. By using the local database containing all drugs on the Belgian market with corresponding active substances, and a pharmacopoeia [34], a complete list of drugs known to influence odor perception was obtained. Where drugs interfering with odor perception did not occur on the list, the person taking them was classified as using "other drugs." Where the person was taking one or more of the drug types on the list, they were classified as using "drugs expected to influence odor perception."

Study Population

Experiment 1

In the first experiment, 67 elderly persons living at home (mean age 66.7 years, SD 6.8, range 55–82) took part. These people all participated in health and fitness programs. All were apparently healthy, without any nasal obstruction and without evidence of acute infection. Participants with alcohol abuse, mental deterioration, and dementia were excluded. Twenty-two used no drugs, 13 used drugs expecting to influence odor perception, and 32 used other drugs, mainly for prophylactic purposes. All participants were independent in the basic activities of daily living.

Experiment 2

Eighty-one persons in retirement homes took part in the second experiment (mean age 82.7 years, SD 7.2, range 61–98). The degree of dependency for basic activities of daily living (ADL) was evaluated with the Katz score [35]. Eleven used no drugs, nine took drugs for prophylactic purposes only, and 61 took drugs expected to influence odor perception. Thirty-five participants were independent, 22 had a minor degree of dependency (score B, C), and 24 participants were highly dependent (score D–G, O).

Statistical Analysis

The equation for the calculation of the sensory detection threshold used for statistical analysis is described by Stevens & Cain [36]. Normal distribution was tested with Kolmogorov-Smirnov test. To test the hypothesis as to whether two group means were equal or not, a Student's *t* test was applied when data were normally distributed. When more than two groups were compared, one-way analysis of variance was used. When two categorical variables were compared, cross-tabulations were used and tested with the χ^2 test. When two continuous variables were compared, Pearson correlation coefficients (r) were calculated and tested for significance. To test the combined contribution of different independent variables on the dependent variable of interest, multiple regression was used. All statistical analysis were conducted using the SPSS package [37].

Results

Experiment 1

Table 1 shows the number of participants living in the community, including their mean age and MNA scores. As illustrated in Figure 2, the correlation between age and MNA score was not significant ($r = 0.03$, $p = 0.39$) and no significant difference was observed in MNA score between men and women (*t* test, $p = 0.12$). A significant correlation was found between age and odor perception ($r = -0.21$, $p < 0.016$), indicating that the proportion of elderly people with a poor

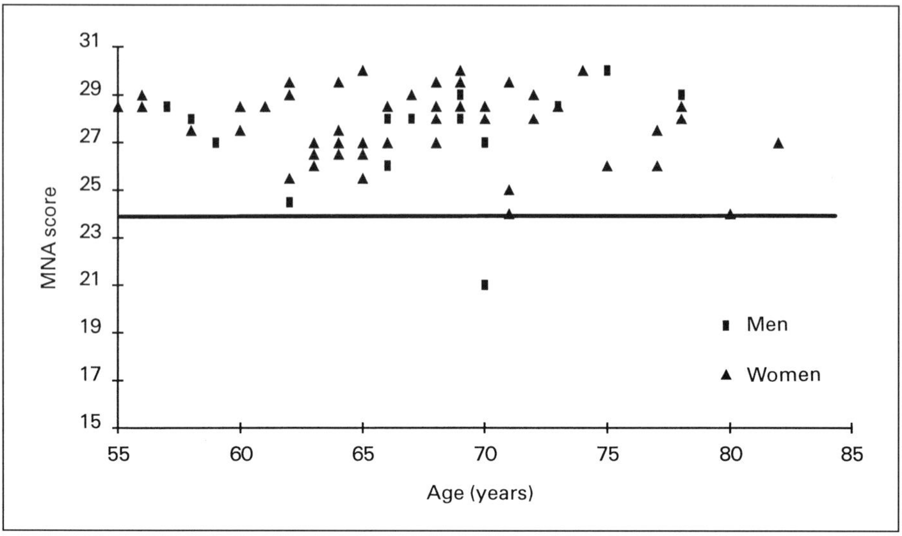

Fig. 2. Age, gender and MNA score of elderly living independently at home (≥24 points = well-nourished, 17–24 points = at risk of malnutrition, <17 points = malnourished).

Table 1. Age and gender distribution of the population living independently at home, with mean Mini Nutritional Assessment (MNA), body mass index (BMI), and Medical Outcome Study (MOS) scores

	Number of persons	Mean BMI kg/m^2 (SD)	Mean age years (SD)	Mean MOS score, % (SD)	Mean MNA score (SD)
Total	67	26.7 (3.9)	66.7 (6.8)	84.1 (12.2)	27.6 (1.7)
Men	15	27.5 (3.9)	66.0 (7.4)	83.9 (12.4)	27.4 (2.1)
Women	52	26.4 (3.9)	66.9 (6.7)	84.2 (12.2)	27.7 (1.6)

sense of smell increases with age. The correlations between age and MOS score ($r = 0.04$, $p = 0.36$), odor perception and MNA score ($r = -0.02$, $p = 0.44$), or odor perception and MOS score ($r = 0.00$, $p = 0.49$) were not significant. However, the MOS score was significantly correlated with the MNA score, showing that a poor state of health status was associated with a high risk of malnutrition ($r = 0.31$, $p = 0.005$ for social functioning; $r = 0.33$, $p = 0.003$ for perceived health). None of the other dimensions showed a significant correlation ($p > 0.05$).

Neither MNA score nor odor perception differed significantly between persons taking drugs affecting odor perception and those taking other types of drugs

Table 2. Age and sex distribution of the population living in retirement homes with mean Mini Nutritional Assessment (MNA), body mass index (BMI), and Medical Outcome Study (MOS) scores

	Number of persons	Mean BMI kg/m^2 (SD)	Mean age years (SD)	Mean MOS score, % (SD)	Mean MNA score (SD)
Total	81	26.4 (4.3)	82.7 (7.2)	62.9 (17.5)	23.6 (2.8)
Men	16	26.8 (3.3)	82.8 (10.4)	71.3 (13.9)	24.6 (2.6)
Women	65	26.3 (4.5)	82.6 (6.3)	60.9 (17.7)	23.4 (2.8)

(*t* test, p = 0.19 and p = 0.96, respectively). Significant correlations were found between age (r = –0.28, p = 0.001), MOS score (r = 0.18, p = 0.039), and number of natural teeth. No significant correlation was observed between number of natural teeth and MNA score (r = 0.01, p = 0.48). None of the anthropometric variables except BMI (r = 0.20, p = 0.05) showed a significant correlation with MNA score ($p > 0.05$).

Among elderly people living independently at home, the effects of age, health status, use of drugs, dental state, body composition, and odor perception can be expected to increase the variability of the MNA score. To test the separate effects of these different independent variables on the risk of malnutrition and to determine their relative importance, multiple regression analysis was used.

The most important variable was AMC, for which there was a significant positive regression coefficient (b = 3.28, p = 0.02), indicating that persons who were not at risk of malnutrition had a higher muscle mass than those with malnutrition (total R^2 = 0.53).

Experiment 2

Table 2 shows the numbers of participants living in retirement homes, with their mean age and MNA scores. As shown in Figure 3, the correlation between age and MNA score was not significant (r = 0.06, p = 0.25). MNA scores for women were significantly lower than for men (p = 0.048). No significant correlation was found between age and odor perception (r = –0.09, p = 0.19). The correlations between age and MOS score (r = –0.14, p = 0.11), and odor perception and MNA score (r = –0.02, p = 0.40) were not significant. However, a high MOS score was associated with good odor perception (r = 0.21, p = 0.03); MOS subscales were also significant: social functioning (r = 0.18, p = 0.04), and mental functioning (r = 0.29, p = 0.003). Significant correlations were found between age and number of natural teeth (r = –0.26, p = 0.001) as well as MNA score and number of natural teeth (r = 0.27, p = 0.001).

MNA scores of people taking drugs affecting odor perception were significantly lower than in those taking other drugs (*t* test, p = 0.001). Neither age nor odor

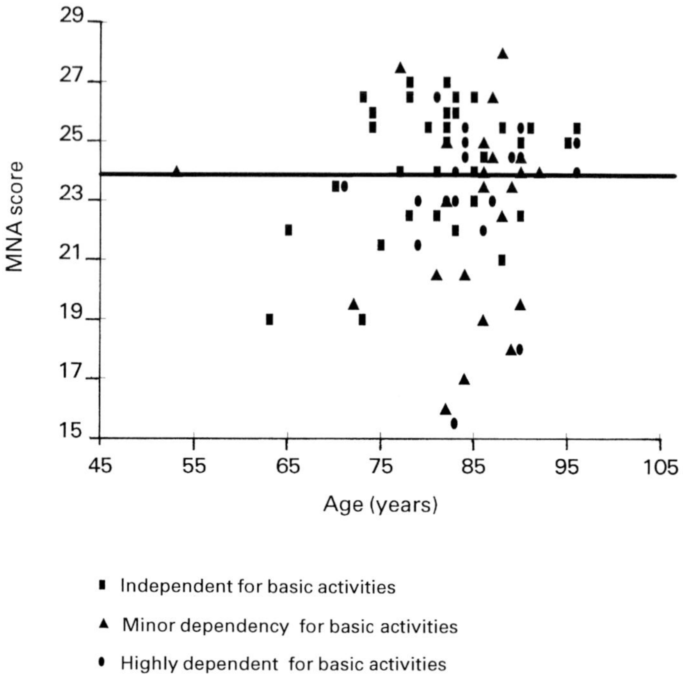

Fig. 3. Age, degree of dependency and MNA score of elderly living in retirement homes ($\geq$24 points = well-nourished, 17–24 points = at risk of malnutrition, <17 points = malnourished).

perception differed significantly between persons taking drugs affecting odor perception and those taking other drugs (*t* test, $p = 0.99$ and $p = 0.42$, respectively).

As can be seen in Table 3, highly significant correlations were found between MNA score and BMI, AMC, AMA ($p < 0.0005$), as well as between MNA score and TST and AFA ($p < 0.05$), indicating that elderly people living in retirement homes who are at risk for malnutrition have lower muscle and fat mass than those not at risk.

To test the separate effects of the different independent variables on the risk of malnutrition and to determine their relative importance, multiple regression analysis was used. The most important variable was health status, showing a significant positive regression coefficient (b = 0.045, $p = 0.05$), implying that persons in a poor state of health are more often at risk of malnutrition than persons in a good health state (total $R^2 = 0.66$).

Table 3. Correlations (p value) between Mini Nutritional Assessment (MNA) and anthropometric measures

	Whole group (n = 148)	Retirement homes (n = 81)	Living at home (n = 67)
BMI, kg/m^2	0.29 (<0.0005)	0.38 (<0.0005)	0.20 (0.05)
Triceps skinfold thickness, mm	0.11 (0.05)	0.28 (<0.0005)	NS
Arm fat area, cm^2	0.14 (0.02)	0.30 (<0.0005)	NS
Arm muscle circumference, cm	0.24 (<0.0005)	0.19 (0.02)	0.18 (0.07)
Arm muscle area, cm^2	0.23 (<0.0005)	0.20 (0.01)	NS
Abdomen/hip ratio	NS	NS	NS

Table 4. Correlations between Medical Outcome Study (MOS) general health scores and Mini Nutritional Assessment (MNA) for male and female elderly people living independently at home and in retirement homes

	Living at home (n = 67)	In retirement homes (n = 81)	Total group (n = 148)
Physical health	NS	NS	0.43 (<0.0005)
Role functioning	NS	NS	0.43 (<0.0005)
Social functioning	0.31 (0.005)	0.18 (0.04)	0.50 (<0.0005)
Mental functioning	NS	0.29 (0.003)	0.42 (<0.0005)
Perceived health	0.33 (0.003)	0.18 (0.18)	0.39 (<0.0005)
Physical pain	NS	NS	NS

Summary of Effects and Comparison between Elderly Living in the Community and Elderly Living in Retirement Homes

Participants living in retirement homes were older than those living in the community ($p < 0.001$). MNA scores for elderly people living in the community were higher than for those living in retirement homes ($p < 0.001$). Only 2% of the elderly people living at home were at risk of malnutrition, compared with 37% of those living in retirement homes ($p < 0.001$). In retirement homes, more people had complete dentures, used drugs affecting odor perception, or had a poor odor perception compared with elderly people living independently at home ($p < 0.001$).

A summary of statistical associations between MNA score and the different age-related phenomena under investigation is given in Tables 3–6 and in Fig-

Table 5. Correlation (*r*) between Mini Nutritional Assessment (MNA) score and indices of sensory perception

	Living at home (n = 67)	In retirement homes (n = 81)	Total group (n = 148)
Odor perception	−0.02 ($p = 0.45$)	0.03 ($p = 0.41$)	0.38* ($p < 0.005$)
Number of natural teeth	0.00 ($p = 0.47$)	0.27* ($p = 0.001$)	0.45* ($p < 0.005$)

* Significant at $p = 0.005$.

Table 6. Mean Mini Nutritional Assessment (MNA) score (SD) and use of drugs affecting odor perception

	Using drugs affecting odor perception	Using other or no drugs
Living at home	26.8 (2.92)	27.8 (1.42)
In retirement homes	23.4* (2.72)	25.5 (1.58)
Whole group	23.8* (2.99)	27.0 (1.83)

* Significant at $p < 0.0005$.

ure 4. In the group as a whole, there was a significant correlation between risk of malnutrition and poor odor perception, as well as between use of drugs that affect odor perception and MNA score. For both elderly people living independently at home and for those living in retirement homes, general health and body composition were important factors, while in retirement homes, the number of natural teeth and the use of drugs are independent factors explaining the risk of malnutrition measured by the MNA score.

Discussion

Many elderly people have a monotonous or inadequate diet and are in a state of marginal nutritional deficiency. Energy intake is often found to be below recommended daily allowances, making it extremely difficult to meet requirements for vitamins and minerals [30, 38, 39]. Deficiencies have been reported for vitamin A, B1, B2, B6, B12, D, folic acid and iron. Malnutrition is associated with

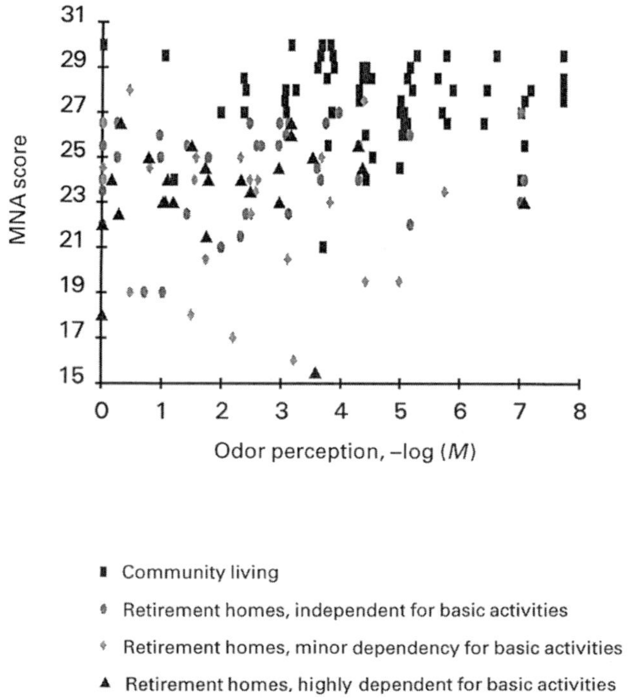

Fig. 4. Odor perception and MNA score ($r = 0.34$, $p < 0.001$).

increased mortality, frailty, increased risk of several diseases, susceptibility to infection, and reduced quality of life [40]. In our study, the risk of malnutrition was evaluated by MNA as a composite measure of 18 nutrition-related items. MNA is a validated quantitative evaluation tool, appropriate for assessing the risk of malnutrition in elderly people. In evaluating odor perception and dental state as a function of nutritional risk, it became clear that the relations between these variables are complex. Among elderly people living at home an association was found between poor general health and a tendency for lower MNA scores. Not surprisingly, persons without risk of malnutrition had a higher muscle mass than those with malnutrition.

Among elderly people living in retirement homes, poor general health was associated with diminished odor perception, and a high risk of malnutrition was associated with a loss of natural teeth. In addition, MNA scores in those taking drugs affecting odor perception were lower than in those taking other drugs.

One would expect a relation between nutritional status and the sense of smell, but the relation between odor perception and nutrition in the elderly is controversial [41]. Poor nutrition with increased risk of several diseases, frailty, and decreased immunity is directly linked with poor general health, affecting sensory capacities. The controversy over the relation between odor perception and nutrition may be the result of the effect of general health and of use of drugs, both of which are linked with both poor nutrition and poor odor perception. The population under investigation was heterogeneous with regard to general health. Many other studies have shown that odor perception is related to medical condition and drug use [2, 13, 14, 25].

Murphy & Whithee [42] found an association between protein status and sensory measures of odor intensity and preference. Mattes *et al.* [12] found no differences in dietary factors (calcium, folic acid and protein), as measured by a food consumption study in patients with smell disorders. Ferris & Duffy [6] conducted a similar study and claimed that the severity of smell dysfunction had an effect on the adequacy of calcium intake. Published reports of the extent and nature of changes in body weight, BMI, and body fat and the relation with smell have also been controversial [41]. Recently, Hunter-Smith & Kessel [43] reported a reciprocal association between the ability to smell and BMI. On the other hand, Duffy *et al.* [10] and Mattes *et al.* [12] reported no differences in energy intake or BMI between those with and without a diminished sense of smell.

Fischer & Johnson [44] suggest that weight loss is multifactorial but can be attributed to diminished odor perception. Along these lines, Mattes *et al.* [12] and Mattes & Coward [45] found that the majority of persons with olfactory disorders show weight loss. Wysocki & Pelchat [14] observed that odor dysfunction can cause loss of enjoyment of eating. Duffy *et al.* [10] found an association between odor/flavor perception and altered preference or consumption of particular foods. A possible explanation could be that a loss of sensations during food consumption accompanies reduced food intake [9].

In general, previous studies where the relation between odor perception and nutritional state was explored did not use composite measures of nutritional risk but focused on single nutritional components, blood chemistries, or anthropometric sites. The MNA is an overall evaluation score of nutritional state and does not provide information about specific nutrients or biochemical indices. The results from previous studies are therefore difficult to compare with MNA scores. In general, focusing on the overall dietary pattern is more important for health, quality of life, and longevity than focusing on individual components [46]. Along these lines, it has been suggested by Mattes & Coward [45] that deficits or excesses of specific nutrients do not explain the age-related abnormalities in taste and smell. Remedies focusing on single nutrients would therefore have limited value.

The MOS scale was used to distinguish the effect of general health from that of odor perception on the variability of nutritional state. In validation studies of the MOS scale carried out by others [29] on a total of 11,186 persons, objective medical data were related to independently obtained MOS scores. It became clear that patients in poor general health, assessed by medical criteria, show on average a 50% lower MOS score than healthy people. People with chronic medical conditions have lower MOS scores than those with acute illnesses or healthy people. These findings indicate that the MOS scale is a useful, reliable, and valid instrument for measuring general health in the elderly.

Our results show a significant relation between nutritional state and general health, while a significant relation was also observed between general health and odor perception. Along these lines, it has been suggested that physiological regression is in general more related to health than to age [47], and health status might also become more important than age for odor perception [9]. However, the results reported in published reports are cross-sectional in nature and do not provide definitive support for the hypothesis that diminished odor perception is caused by poor health or that improvement of general health might improve odor perception.

Volatile odors, originating from food, enter the nasal cavity retronasally during mastication. Decreased chewing ability in elderly people may prevent the release of the odors from the food. Decreased appetite and decreased ability to eat can restrict food selection [48], leading to poor nutrition. Papas *et al.* [20] showed a 20% drop in nutritional quality of food consumed by people who had upper or lower dentures, or both, compared with those who had their natural teeth. The chewing ability of denture wearers is particularly reduced, so they often choose only soft food, which frequently is nutritionally unbalanced [22, 49]. People wearing complete dentures have one sixth the masticatory ability of those with their natural dentition [50]. Tooth loss causes a significant loss of chewing ability, and complete dentures do not restore full oral function. Impaired mastication alters the sensory and psychological aspects of eating, causing restriction of food selection. Recent population-based studies suggest that edentulousness is correlated with reduced nutrient intakes and multiple dietary inadequacies, and edentulous individuals are more likely to have an atherogenic diet [19]. Our results with MNA show that the risk of malnutrition increases with tooth loss and with wearing complete dentures. Owing to the cross-sectional nature of our data, the results show no causal effect of dental state. Dental state may not be a direct cause of malnutrition but a contributing factor in those elderly people who have other risk factors [48].

In conclusion, our results show that elderly people at risk of malnutrition tend to have poorer health, poorer odor perception, and fewer natural teeth than elderly people not at risk of malnutrition.

Part 2

Malnutrition and Flavor Amplification

In part 1, it became clear that with age, poor nutritional status, and poor health status, odor perception declines to a considerable extend. On a group level, elderly people at risk of malnutrition tend to have worse odor perception than those not at risk of malnutrition. Since food flavors consist mainly of volatile odors, and flavor perception has been rated as the strongest determinant of food choice in the elderly [15], in this study we examined whether increasing the flavor level of food improved food preference and consumption of elderly people at risk of malnutrition.

Compensating for diminished sensory function with age might improve the quality of life for elderly people. Previous studies have shown that flavor amplification improves both preference and consumption of particular foods [31, 51, 52]. Since food habits of many elderly people are inadequate, leading to a poor nutritional state, nutrient-dense foods are the prime candidates for flavor amplification. Adding odors to nutrient-dense foods might act to make food more appealing and increase consumption in elderly people in a poor nutritional state. Compared with (saturated) fat, sugar and salt, exposure to additional amounts of flavors is generally harmless and self-limiting, with no detrimental health effects since only small quantities – well below the maximal tolerable doses – are needed to give foods a perceptibly stronger flavor [2].

For its nutritional benefit, it was decided in this study to test whether flavor amplification induced changes in preference and consumption of skimmed yogurt, and whether elderly people in a poor nutritional state could benefit from this.

Subjects and Methods

The study populations were the same as in experiments 1 and 2 of part 1 (Tables 1 and 2).

Food System for Flavor Amplification

Skimmed yoghurt was chosen as a major source of calcium and for its potential beneficial effects on cholesterol balance, cancer prevention, and immune function [53, 54].

The optimal sensory quality of the yoghurt was assessed during extended pilot studies with equal flavor intensities. The concentration ranges of flavors in the food samples were assessed by scientists of Perlarom S.A. (Belgium). All flavors used were mixtures of odoriferous molecules extracted from natural products or synthesized after chemical analysis of the natural product. Obvious differences between high and low concentrations of flavor in the samples were created for odoriferous compounds only, while preparation and logistical procedures were standardized. The other sensory characteristics such as taste, color, and texture were held constant.

For the preparation of the yoghurt samples, 25.0 g simplex sugar syrup (Pharmacopoeia) was mixed with 0.200 or 1.000 ml strawberry flavor (Perlarom S.A., Belgium) for low and high flavor levels, respectively; 375.0 g skimmed yoghurt (Delhaize, Belgium) was mixed with the syrup until the mixture was homogeneous.

Preference and Consumption Measurements

In random order, participants received two food samples (20 g) in small identical cups, pairwise at the same time, one containing the high food flavor level and the other the low flavor level. Participants were asked to indicate whether they could taste a difference between the food samples and if so, which of the two they preferred. The ratings were checked by the qualitative reactions of the participants.

During 2 days, independent of the preference measures, food dishes were supplied to the participants under controlled conditions between meals. In random order, participants received 400 g yoghurt with either a high or low flavor level. Sufficient food was available to allow respondents to eat as much as they wanted to, thus allowing consumption levels to be compared. On each testing day, all dishes were prepared individually under the same conditions. Participants were ignorant of the details of the study and it was verified that they added no sugar or other substances to the yoghurt. To measure the differences in consumed quantities, portions were weighed before and after the session. Testing took place in clean, ventilated, neutral dining rooms that were used for this experiment only and free of smoke or loud noise. Testing days were carefully selected by consulting the management of the centers to make sure that the meals supplied on both testing days were comparable in terms of energy contents and serving time. Before the sessions, the subjects were interviewed to verify that they did not consume either excessive or minimal amounts during their meals. If they did, they were excluded from further statistical analysis.

Results

Table 7 shows the mean MNA scores and ages of the elderly people preferring a high or a low flavor level. The proportion of men and women preferring either flavor level was equally distributed (χ^2 test, $p > 0.11$). Among elderly people living

Table 7. Mini Nutritional Assessment (MNA) score, age, and preference for flavor-amplified food

	Total group	At home	In retirement homes
Preference for low flavor			
Mean MNA score (SD)	25.8* (2.6)	27.5 (1.9)	24.4* (2.3)
Mean age, years (SD)	73.7 (10.9)	65.2* (6.2)	83.7 (5.3)
Preference for high flavor			
Mean MNA score (SD)	24.6 (3.5)	27.7 (1.7)	22.9 (3.0)
Mean age, years (SD)	76.6 (10.2)	68.0 (6.6)	83.7 (6.4)

* Significant difference between persons preferring high and low odor level ($p < 0.05$).

Table 8. Nutritional risk in relation to flavor amplification, correlations between Mini Nutritional Assessment (MNA) score and consumed quantities of flavor-amplified yogurt (p value)

	High flavor level yogurt	Low flavor level yogurt
Total group (n = 148)	0.13 (0.054)	0.26 (0.001)*
Elderly people in retirement homes (n = 81)	0.09 (0.18)	0.14 (0.08)
Elderly people at home (n = 67)	0.07 (0.32)	0.04 (0.41)

* Significant at $p = 0.001$.

independently at home, no significant difference was observed in MNA score between those preferring a high and those preferring a low flavor level; however, those preferring a high flavor level were significantly older than those preferring a low flavor level (t test, $p < 0.05$).

Elderly people in retirement homes preferring the high strawberry flavor level had significantly lower MNA scores than those preferring the low flavor level (t test, $p < 0.05$). No significant difference in age was observed between those preferring high and low flavor levels.

A highly significant correlation was observed between the consumption of low flavor level yogurt and MNA score ($r = 0.26$, $p = 0.001$), indicating that elderly subjects at risk of malnutrition consume less of the low flavor level yogurt. No significant correlation was observed between consumption of the high flavor level yoghurt and MNA score ($r = 0.13$, $p = 0.054$; Table 8).

A combined effect of age and MNA score on consumption levels is to be expected, so multiple regression analysis was used to determine their relative importance. Regression coefficients for both age and MNA score were significant ($p = 0.02$), showing that the effects of MNA and age on consumption levels are independent – for example, the effect of the MNA score cannot be ascribed to age (total $R^2 = 0.31$).

Discussion and Conclusion

Elderly people suffering from malnutrition might benefit from flavor-amplified food, and our results confirm that flavor amplification can influence food preference [31]. Compared to relatively young persons, most elderly people reacted positively to the flavor-amplified food and preferred high flavor levels. Elderly people who preferred a high strawberry flavor level tended to have lower MNA scores than those who preferred a low flavor level. In addition, a low MNA score was associated with a reduced consumption of low flavor level food, while the consumption of flavor-amplified food remained constant when the MNA score was low. Therefore, in order to assure that consumption levels of elderly people suffering from malnutrition remain the same as in well-nourished elderly people, flavor amplification is necessary and is generally harmless compared with adding fat, salt, and sugar.

However, caution is required, since the results are based only on 2 days of meal supply under controlled conditions and in selected elderly populations. Our results do not show whether improved preference would continue after 2 days, or whether they can be generalized to a larger range of candidate food products for flavor amplification. The aged population is heterogeneous in terms of health status, sensory capacities, nutritional state, living conditions, functional ability, attitudes, and perceived risk [55]. Therefore, the acceptability of flavor-amplified food for consumers under real-life conditions, including additional factors that determine food choice, deserves further study [52].

References

1. Doty RL. Psychophysical measurement of odor perception in humans. In: Laing DG, Doty RL, Breipohl W, eds. *The human sense of smell.* Berlin: Springer Verlag, 1991: 95–135.
2. Schiffman S. Olfaction in aging and medical disorders. In: Serby MJ, Chobor KL, eds. *Science of olfaction.* New York: Springer Verlag, 1992: 500–26.
3. Wysocki CJ, Gilbert AN. National Geographic smell survey: effects of age are heterogeneous. *Ann NY Acad Sci* 1989; 561: 12–29.
4. Schiffman S. Age related changes in taste and smell and their possible causes. In: Meiselman HL, Rivlin RS, eds. *Clinical measurement of taste and smell.* New York: Macmillan, 1986: 325–42.
5. Chauhan J, Hawrysh ZJ, Gee M, Donald EA, Basu TK. Age-related olfactory and taste changes and interrelations between taste and nutrition. *J Am Diet Assoc* 1987; 87: 1543–51.
6. Ferris AM, Duffy VB. Effect of olfactory deficits on nutritional status: does age predict a person at risk? *Ann NY Acad Sci* 1989; 561: 76–87.

7. Murphy C. Age-associated changes in taste and odor sensations, perception and preference. In: Munro H, Schlierf G, eds. *Nutrition of the elderly.* New York: Raven Press, 1992: 78–89.
8. Guigoz Y, Vellas B, Garry PJ. Assessing the nutritional status of elderly. *Nutr Rev* 1996; 54: S59–65.
9. Griep MI, Mets TF, Vercruysse A, *et al.* Food odor thresholds in relation with age, nutritional and health status. *J Gerontol* 1995; 503; B407–14.
10. Duffy VB, Backstrand JR, Ferris AM. Olfactory dysfunction and related nutritional risk in free-living, elderly women. *J Am Diet Assoc* 1995; 95: 879–84.
11. Schiffman S, Warwick ZS. Changes in taste and smell over the life span: effects on appetite and nutrition in the elderly. In: Friedman MI, Tordoff ME, Kare MR, eds. *Chemical senses.* New York: Marcel Dekker, 1991: 341–65.
12. Mattes RD, Coward BJ, Schiavo MA, *et al.* Dietary evaluations of patients with smell and/or taste disorders. *Am J Clin Nutr* 1990; 51: 233–40.
13. Griep MI, Mets TF, Collys K, Vogelaere P, Laska M, Massart DL. Odor perception in relation to age, general health, anthropometry and dental state. *Arch Gerontol Geriatr* 1997; 25: 263–75.
14. Wysocki CJ, Pelchat ML. The effects of aging on the human sense of smell and its relationship to food choice. *Crit Rev Food Sci Nutr* 1993; 33: 63–82.
15. Rolls BJ. Aging and appetite. *Nutr Rev* 1992; 50: 422–6.
16. Sugano H. Psychophysiological studies of fragrances. In: van Toller S, Dodd GH, eds. *Fragrance, the psychology and biology of perfume.* London: Elsevier, 1992: 221–9.
17. de Baat C, Kalk W, Schuil GRE. The effectiveness of oral hygiene programmes for elderly people – a review. *Gerodontology* 1993; 10: 109–13.
18. Rolls BJ. Appetite and satiety in the elderly. *Nutr Rev* 1994; 52: S9–10.
19. Shay KS, Ship JA. The importance of oral health in the older patient. *J Am Geriatr Soc* 1995; 43: 1414–22.
20. Papas AS, Palmer CA, Rounds MC. Longitudinal relationships between nutrition and oral health. *Ann NY Acad Sci* 1989; 561: 124–43.
21. Touyz LZ. Oral malodor – a review. *J Can Dent Assoc* 1993; 59: 607–10.
22. Horwath CC. Dietary intake studies in elderly people. *World Rev Nutr Diet* 1989; 59: 1–70.
23. Griep MI, Verleye G, Mets TF, Massart DL. Variation in nutrient intake with dental status, age and odor perception. *Eur J Clin Nutr* 1996; 50: 816–25.
24. Cain WS, Gent JF. Olfactory sensitivity: reliability, generality, and association with aging. *J Exp Psychol Hum Percept Perform* 1992; 17: 382–91.
25. Doty RL, Kobal G. Current trends in the measurements of olfactory function. In: Doty RL, ed. *Handbook of olfaction and gustation.* New York: Marcel Dekker, 1995: 191–225.
26. Laska M, Hudson RA. Comparison of the detection threshold of odor mixtures and their components. *Chem Senses* 1991; 16: 651–63.
27. Devos M, Patte F, Rouault J. *Standardized human olfactory thresholds.* New York: IRL Press, 1990.
28. Guigoz Y, Vellas B, Garry PJ. Mini nutritional assessment: a practical tool for grading the nutritional state of elderly patients. *Facts Res Gerontol* 1994 (suppl): 15–61.
29. Stewart AL, Greenfield S, Hays RD, *et al.* Functional status and well-being of patients with chronic conditions. *JAMA* 1989; 262: 907–13.
30. Shils ME, Olson JA, Shike M. *Modern nutrition in health and disease,* 8th ed. Philadelphia: Lea & Febiger, 1994.
31. Schiffman S, Warwick ZS. Effect of flavor enhancement of foods for the elderly on nutritional state: food intake, biochemical indices and anthropometric measures. *Physiol Behav* 1993; 53: 395–402.
32. Doty RL, Bartoshuk LM, Snow JB. Causes of olfactory and gustatory disorders. In: Getchell ML, Doty RL, Bartoshuk LM, Snow JB, eds. *Smell and taste in health and disease,* 8th ed. New York: Raven Press, 1991.
33. Ship JA, Pearson JD, Cruise LJ, Brant LJ, Metter EJ. Longitudinal changes in smell identification. *J Gerontol* 1996; 51A: M86–91.
34. Reynolds JEF. *Martindale, the extra pharmacopoeia.* London: The Pharmaceutical Press, 1993.
35. Katz S, Ford AB, Moskowitz RW, *et al.* The index of ADL: a standardised measure of biological and psychological function. *JAMA* 1963; 185: 914–9.
36. Stevens JC, Cain WS. Old-age deficits in the sense of smell as gauged by magnitude matching, and odor identification. *Psychol Aging* 1987; 2: 36–42.
37. SPSS Inc. *User guide SPSS/PC+ Statistics 4.0.* Gorinchem: SPSS International BV, 1990.
38. Silver AJ. Anorexia of aging and protein-energy malnutrition. In: Morley JE, Glick Z, Rubenstein LZ, eds. *Geriatric nutrition, a comprehensive review.* New York: Raven Press, 1990: 105–17.

39. de Groot LPGM, Hautvast JGAJ, van Staveren WA. Nutrition and health of elderly people in Europe: the Euronut-Seneca study. *Nutr Rev* 1992; 50: 185–94.
40. Steen B. Practical aspects of nutrition of the elderly in institutions. In: Munro H, Schlierf G, eds. *Nutrition of the elderly.* New York: Raven Press, 1992: 211–17.
41. Friedman MI, Mattes RD. Chemical senses and nutrition. In: Getchell ML, Doty RL, Bartoshuk LM, Snow JB, eds. *Smell and taste in health and disease,* 8th ed. New York: Raven press, 1991: 391–405.
42. Murphy C, Whithee J. Age and biochemical status predict preference for casein hydrolysate. *J Gerontol* 1987; 42: 73–7.
43. Hunter-Smith DG, Kessel K. Association between elevated body-mass index and impaired sense of smell in older people. *J Am Geriatr Soc* 1996; 44: 100–1.
44. Fischer J, Johnson MA. Low body weight and weight loss in the aged. *J Am Diet Assoc* 1990; 90: 1697–706.
45. Mattes RD, Coward BJ. Dietary intake of patients with chemosensory disorders. *J Am Diet Assoc* 1994; 94: 50–6.
46. Trichopoulou A, Kouris-Blazos A, Wahlqvist ML, *et al.* Diet and overall survival in elderly people. *BMJ* 1995; 311: 1457–60.
47. Briley ME. Food preferences of the elderly. *Nutr Rev* 1994; 52: S21–3.
48. Kaurich M. The oral cavity and nutrition. In: Morley JE, Glick Z, Rubenstein LZ, eds. *Geriatric nutrition, a comprehensive review.* New York: Raven Press, 1990: 225–31.
49. Nagao M. The effects of aging on mastication. *Nutr Rev* 1992; 50: 434–8.
50. Kapur KK, Soman SD. Masticatory performance and efficiency in dental wearers. *J Prosth Dent* 1964; 14: 687–94.
51. Schiffman S, Warwick ZS. Use of flavor-amplified foods to improve nutritional status in the elderly. *Ann NY Acad Sci* 1989; 561: 267–77.
52. Griep MI, Mets TF, Massart DL. Different effects of flavor amplification of nutrient dense foods on preference and consumption in young and elderly subjects. *Food Qual Prefer* 1997; 8: 151–6.
53. Rafter JJ. The role of lactic acid bacteria in colon cancer prevention. *Scand J Gastroenterol* 1995; 30: 497–502.
54. Schiffrin EJ, Rochat F, Link-Amster H, Aeschlimann JM, Donnet-Hughes A. Immunomodulation of human blood cells following the ingestion of lactic acid bacteria. *J Dairy Sci* 1995; 76: 1819–28.
55. Rozin P. The role of learning in the acquisition of food preferences by humans. In: Shepherd R, ed. *Handbook of the psychophysiology of human eating.* Chichester: John Wiley, 1989: 205–31.

Discussion

Dr. Rubenstein: All three papers made some important points. The question I have concerns all three of them. Dr. Griep, on your last slide with your conclusions, the information you presented was really a hypothesis rather than a set of conclusions, and it needs to be established that people who are at risk of malnutrition may benefit from enhanced flavor. Again, there are definite correlations between low scores on the MNA and, for example, low T cell function and mortality. These are important correlations, but they imply the need for interventional studies. We don't know how much of the correlation is due to the malnutrition itself and how much to comorbidity. My feeling is that a significant amount of the correlation is due to the malnutrition, but not all of it. We need to be cautious about how we state these correlations; they set the stage for future interventional trials where we take the people who are clearly at risk for malnutrition or who have low MNA scores and do an intervention.

Dr. Griep: At the Faculty of Medicine and Pharmacy in Brussels, we have just started such an intervention, and we are now testing whether flavor amplification leads to a long-term effect.

Dr. Guesry: Did you measure zinc status in your patients? There are old papers that mention that flavor perception is related to zinc deficiency.

Dr. Griep: We measured plasma zinc and none of the subjects had a low zinc level. This is one of the points that I discussed in my PhD thesis: the relation between zinc status and sensory perception has indeed been described in the literature, but I could not confirm that any specific nutrient showed a clear relation with declining sensory perception. That was one of the reasons why I started working with MNA – I was expecting MNA to be a composite measure, a global score reflecting more than a single nutrient.

Dr. Eastwood: There appeared to be no correlation between MNA scores and the odor perception threshold in people living in the community – as I understood it – nor for people in institutions. But you did get a fit if you put them together. So essentially, you had two groups of people. If you look at the scattergram, it's not really very convincing. What do you think?

Dr. Griep: I agree. The relation *is* there, but becomes much weaker if you split the groups.

Mini Nutritional Assessment (MNA): Research and Practice in the Elderly.
B. Vellas; P.J. Garry; Y. Guigoz (eds),
Nestlé Nutrition Workshop Series Clinical & Performance Programme, Vol. 1, pp. 61–66,
Nestec Ltd.; Vevey/S. Karger AG, Basel, © 1999.

The MNA Score in People Who Have Aged Successfully

K. Scheirlinckx, B. Vellas[a] and P.J. Garry[b]

Clinique Universitaire de Mont-Godinne, Yvoir, Belgium;
[a] Department of Internal Medicine and Clinical Gerontology, CHU Purpan, Toulouse, France;
and [b] New Mexico Aging Process Study, Albuquerque, N.M., USA

One of the main objectives of gerontological medicine is to assist people reaching retirement age to age successfully. As defined by Rowe & Khan [1, 2], successful aging encompasses three distinct domains: avoidance of disease and disability; maintenance of high physical and cognitive function, and sustained engagement in social and productive activities. More studies are needed which contrast successful aging with unsuccessful aging or with pathological conditions leading to poor health status. These studies will enable clinicians to become more aware of how to maintain or restore an acceptable degree of health to elderly patients.

Studies designed to examine the impact of good nutritional habits in maintaining the health status of elderly people have shown that assessing the degree of undernutrition in an elderly patient can be beneficial in the treatment of that patient [3, 4]. However, until recently there has not been a reliable, validated instrument to assess whether poor nutritional habits may be the cause of poor health or may possibly impede the restoration of good health in some elderly patients. The Mini Nutritional Assessment (MNA) was designed for this purpose. The MNA [5] is a standardized and validated instrument which can be easily administered in a short period of time to determine whether the patient may be at risk for undernutrition. In this chapter, we describe the results of using the MNA instrument in 330 elderly individuals enrolled in the New Mexico Aging Process Study (NMAPS) [6].

Materials and Methods

The NMAPS is a longitudinal, multidisciplinary investigation of age-related changes in nutritional status in relation to health and functional status of an elderly cohort. The characteristics and general inclusion criteria for the study are

Table 1. Description of the population studied in 1993

Number	330
Male	132 (40%)
Female	198 (60%)
Age	76.9 ± 6.4
Male	77.0 ± 5.8
Female	76.9 ± 6.7

Table 2. Four stage classification of the participants by health status and by disease (1990)

Classification 1 (C1) Excellent	Classification 2 (C2) Good	Classification 3 (C3) Frail	Classification 4 (C4) Sick
No history of medical or surgical illness	< 2 major medical illness or surgery	Many illness or surgeries	Many major illnesses or surgeries
No HBP or hypothyroidism	Maybe HBP or hypothyroidism		
No significant medications	Few medications	Several significant medications	Many significant medications
Minimal balance or gait abnormalities	1 or 2 balance and gait abnormalities	Many balance or gait abnormalities	Major balance and gait abnormalities
MMS > 27	MMS > 27	MMS < 27	MMS < 25
No deficit in IADL	1 or 2 deficits in IADL	Several IADL deficiencies	Dependent in most IADL

MMS = Mini-mental state examination score; HBP = high blood pressure; IADL = independent activities of daily living.

described elsewhere [6]. It should be noted that the NMAPS is not a "representative" or "population-based" sample, but a cohort of independently living, relatively healthy, economically secure, well-educated, and highly cooperative elderly men and women. Table 1 describes the cohort examined in 1993.

A four-stage classification that defines the state of health of the elderly in the NMAPS was used for this study. The criteria used for this classification were medical history (defined major illnesses, previous major surgery resulting in disability, and present use of drug treatments), gait and balance disorders [7], and cognitive function (mini-mental state (MMSE) score) [8]. Health classification was as follows: C1 = excellent, C2 = good, C3 = frail, C4 = sick (Table 2). In

Table 3. Distribution over the different classes

	Excellent (C1)	Good (C2)	Frail (C3)	Sick (C4)
Number	79 (23.9%)	159 (48.2%)	61 (18.5%)	31 (9.4%)
Age (years)	74.4±5.7	76.3±6.07	9.9±6.6	80.5±6.0
Male	33 (25.0%)	61 (46.2%)	22 (16.7%)	16 (12.1%)
Female	46 (23.2%)	98 (49.5%)	39 (19.7%)	15 (7.6%)

Table 4. Mini-Nutritional Assessment (MNA) scores and serum albumin concentrations

	C1	C2	C3	C4
MNA (max. 30 pts)	27.7±1.8	26.6±2.2	25.7±2.5	24.8±2.8
Albumin (g/l)	41.2±2.3	41.2±2.7	41.0±2.4	39.8±2.9

addition, other information from the NMAPS participants, collected as part of routine yearly measurements, was also available, for example an assortment of biochemical tests. The MNA was administered to all of the NMAPS participants in 1993.

Statistical Analysis

We use analysis of variance to test for differences between groups in means of continuous variables, and the χ^2 test for group differences in frequencies for categorical variables. A probability (p) value of < 0.05 was considered significant.

Results

Table 3 shows the distribution of the four health classifications of the NMAPS participants by sex, along with mean ages in each classification. The highest percentage of participants was classified as being in good health (C2). We found that 72.2% of this cohort were either in good or excellent health by our classification. Mean age increased significantly from C1 to C4 as expected. No significant sex differences were found in any of the health classification categories.

Table 4 shows the mean MNA scores and standard deviations by health classification, along with serum albumin concentrations. The mean MNA score decreased significantly ($p < 0.05$) between those in excellent health status (C1) and those found to be sick (C4). Though mean serum albumin concentrations

Table 5. Good and excellent health versus frail and sick health

	C1 + C2 (72%) (n = 238)	C3 + C4 (28%) (n = 92)	ANOVA
Age (years)	75.7	80.1	$p = 0.0001$
MNA (max. 30 pts)	27.0±2.1	25.4±2.4	$p = 0.0001$
BMI (kg/m^2	25.2	25.2	$p = 0.9172$
Albumin (g/l)	41.2±2.5	40.7±2.1	$p = 0.1016$

were lower in the C4 category compared with the other three categories, this decrease was not statistically significant. A much clearer differentiation between health status and MNA score was found when we grouped those in excellent or good health together (C1 + C2) and compared them with those in the frail or sick category (C3 + C4; Table 5). Seventy-two percent of the participants in the NMAPS were defined as being in good or excellent health (C1 + C2) and 28% were found to be frail or sick (C3 + C4). There were significant differences between these two groups in age and MNA.

Discussion

Rowe & Khan [1, 2] pointed out the need to distinguish "usual" aging (non-disabled older persons: a non-pathologic but high-risk population, meaning there are age-related alterations in functional or cognitive status) from the "successful aging" (that is, people with a low probability of disease and disease-related disability, good functional and cognitive status, and active engagement in life). By this distinction, Rowe & Khan hope to stimulate research into the criteria and determinants of successful aging and identify proper targets for intervention to attain more successful aging in elderly people.

In recent years, successful aging has become a familiar term among gerontologists [9–13]. Geriatric assessment appears useful in describing the successful aging process. The relation between nutritional status and aging has been a subject of growing interest for many years and now we have improved our knowledge on the nutritional needs of elderly people. In the present study, we determined MNA scores in the MNAPS population (n = 330), which we judged was primarily aging successfully – that is, it was mainly composed of those in good or excellent health for their age. The mean (SD) MNA score was significantly higher for those in good and excellent health compared with those judged to be frail or sick: 27.0 (2.1) *vs.* 25.4 (2.6), respectively. The body mass index and albumin values were similar between the two groups.

Conclusions

We consider that an MNA score of < 17 reflects protein-energy malnutrition, a score between 17 and 23.5 reflects risk of malnutrition, and >24 reflects good nutritional status for the elderly population. From our study, an MNA score of around 27 (2.1) seems to be related to successful aging, but more studies are needed to confirm this observation. Maybe this score of 27/30 is one of the criteria which should be present, among others, for the definition of a successful aging process.

References

1. Rowe JW, Khan RL. Human aging: usual and successful. *Science* 1987; 237: 143–9.
2. Rowe JW, Khan RL. Successful aging. *Gerontologist* 1997; 37: 433–40.
3. Hartz SC, *et al. Nutrition in the elderly: the Boston Nutritional Status Survey.* London: Smith-Gordon-Nishiruma, 1989.
4. Harris T, Burt V, Hitchcock D, Maurer K. The National Health and Nutrition Examination Survey III (NHANES III): contributions to the study of aging and aged. *Année Gérontol* 1990; 4: 317–21.
5. Vellas B, Guigoz Y, Garry PI, Albarede JL. *The Mini Nutritional Assessment, MNA.* Paris: Editions Serdi, 1995.
6. Garry PJ, Owen MO, Eldidge TO. *The New Mexico Aging Process Study.* Albuquerque: Clinical Nutrition Programme, University of New Mexico, 1997.
7. Tinetti ME, Speechley M, Ginter SF. Risk factors for falls among elderly persons living in the community. *N Engl J Med* 1988; 319: 1701–7.
8. Folstein ME, Folstein SE, McHugh PR. "Mini Mental State": a practical guide for grading the cognitive state of patients for the clinicians. *J Psychiatr Res* 1975; 12: 189–98.
9. Abeles RP, Gift HC, Ory MG. *Aging and quality of life.* New York: Springer, 1994; 185–205.
10. Baltes MM, Baltes PB. *Successful aging: perspective from the behavioral sciences.* Cambridge: Cambridge University Press, 1994.
11. Garfein AJ, Hergoz AR. Robust aging among the young-old, old-old and oldest-old. *J Gerontol B Psychol Sci Soc Sci* 1995; 50: S77–87.
12. Butter RN, Gleason HP. *Productive aging enhancing vitality in later life.* New York: Springer, 1985.
13. Berkman LF, Seeman TE, Albert MA, Blazer D, Kahn R, Mohs R, *et al.* High, usual and impaired functioning in community dwelling older men and women: findings from the MacArthur Foundation research network on successful aging. *J Clin Epidemiolol* 1993; 46: 1129–40.
14. *Health. United States, 1989.* Hyattsville, Maryland: National Center for Health Statistics, 1990.

Discussion

Dr. Camilla: If I understood you correctly, your study was a longitudinal one, although I believe you presented cross-sectional data. I think it is important for a successful evaluation of aging in relation to MNA to have information on lifestyle factors, including dietary habits. Could you comment on that?

Dr. Scheirlinckx: We did make a cross-sectional analysis in 1993 but I have no information on lifestyle factors.

Dr. Vellas: The aim of the study was only to obtain MNA scores in healthy elderly people. We know that the MNA score is around 27–28 in these people. Maybe this would be a suitable goal for people who age successfully.

Dr. Rea: I am still concerned about the MNA values in healthy old people. In our over-90 population – which is presumably composed of people who have aged successfully, since they have managed to reach that great age – our MNA scores were 23 for females and

24 for males. It does worry me that you're thinking in terms of scores of 27 or 28 in successful aging. Our experience is that the scores are a good deal lower than that.

Dr. Vellas: I don't think that reaching the age of 90 is equivalent to successful aging. You can be 90 years old and frail. It would be important to have a full geriatric assessment in your population and to select only the 90-year-olds who are in good health as opposed to those who are really frail and see what the MNA score is in them. I expect your population includes people with gait and balance disorders, people on drug treatment, and people with diseases of various kinds.

Dr. Rea: If you look at our poster, you will find that there was only one person who was not able to walk independently.

Dr. Vellas: Yes, but walking independently does not rule out frailty. Are you sure your subjects were not on medication, and had no gait or balance disorder, or cognitive impairment?

Dr. Rea: Our population has no cognitive impairment, they have virtually no gait disturbance, and they are apparently healthy, although they are on drugs. About a third of them would be taking medication. I would argue that they have successfully aged. They may be frail, but they have successfully aged.

Dr. Chumlea: I think what Dr. Rea is bringing up is an interesting question. There does seem to be an age effect, with older people having a smaller MNA score. So there is confounding here that maybe needs to be corrected for, though I don't know exactly how to do it.

Dr. Morley: I think the problem is how you define successful aging. There are clearly highly successful, highly functional people in the 90+ age range, who are still capable of doing things that many of us have never done or never even conceived we could do. These are the people who are truly successful at aging. Another group is the people who have diseases and are somewhat frail but are coping, and because they are coping they are getting to an older age. I don't think of them as truly successful at aging. They have overcome problems, and they are living with problems. We have lots of 90-year-olds functioning fairly well in the community, but many are very frail. We need to know whether the people in the Irish group with low MNA scores have greater morbidity over period of time and die sooner than those who score higher. Only when we have those data will we be able to determine who are the truly successful ones.

Dr. Chumlea: I agree that a score of between 17 and 23 places the individual at risk, and may have important significance in people of 70–85. But once you get to 95 it's impossible to have a score as high as 27. It's bound to be depressed because of frailties. That does not mean that such people are not aging successfully, but there will be a decline with age which needs to be taken account of in the score.

Dr. Vellas: For this reason I think that 23.5 for a 90-year-old is not such a bad score. It's the same as with the Mini Mental State score. If we look at people over 90, sometimes some of them can have a score of 26 or 27 on the MMS.

Dr. Rea: Our group were all over 28, and most of them 30. They are not mentally impaired.

Dr. Rubenstein: This discussion illustrates the importance of not relying on a number *per se* in all these screening tests. They are simply screening tests. The crucial thing is that when you notice a discrepancy between a score and what you think is happening clinically, you look at what the scale is actually saying. What are the items that are responsible for this fall off? Are they an age-related phenomenon, or a cultural difference? Is there something different about Ireland – or maybe something different about people in their 90s – that is pulling down the score? Is it only one or two items on the MNA? You need to look at those items rather than simply taking the number *per se.*

Dr. Vellas: We do know that people who are over 90 are at risk of malnutrition if they have some kind of disease.

Mini Nutritional Assessment (MNA): Research and Practice in the Elderly:
B. Vellas; P.J. Garry; Y. Guigoz (eds),
Nestlé Nutrition Workshop Series Clinical & Performance Programme, Vol. 1, pp. 67–77,
Nestec Ltd.; Vevey/S. Karger AG, Basel, © 1999.

Anorexia of Aging, Leptin, and the Mini Nutritional Assessment

J.E. Morley, D.K. Miller, H.M. Perry III, P. Patrick, Y. Guigoz[b] and B. Vellas[a]

GRECC, St. Louis VAMC, and Division of Geriatric Medicine, Saint Louis University, Saint Louis, Mo., USA; [a] University of Toulouse, France; [b] Nestlé Research Center, Nestec Ltd., Lausanne, Switzerland

It is now well established that there is a linear decrease in food intake of humans over the life span [1]. This occurs in the face of an increase in weight and body fat in middle age. This conundrum suggests that the increase in weight at middle age is not caused by alterations in food intake but rather by changes in physical activity, metabolic rate, or efficiency at laying down adipose tissue. In this chapter we will first review the pathophysiological mechanisms associated with the development of the anorexia of aging and then briefly review the causes of malnutrition in older persons. In the final two sections we provide new data on the relation of leptin to the Mini Nutritional Assessment (MNA) and the relation of the MNA to malnutrition in an older, free-living, inner city African American population.

Anorexia of Aging

Dysregulation of food intake in healthy elderly people has been clearly shown [2, 3]. Roberts *et al.* [2] found that when older persons were either underfed or overfed, they were less capable of altering their food intake to return their weight to premanipulation levels. Wurtman *et al.* [3] showed that healthy older people ingest less food than younger people and that this is predominantly due to a reduction in fat intake. In our studies we have found that older persons have a greater degree of satiation following a standard meal than younger persons [4]. Older people have a delay in gastric emptying and this is related to the degree of hunger

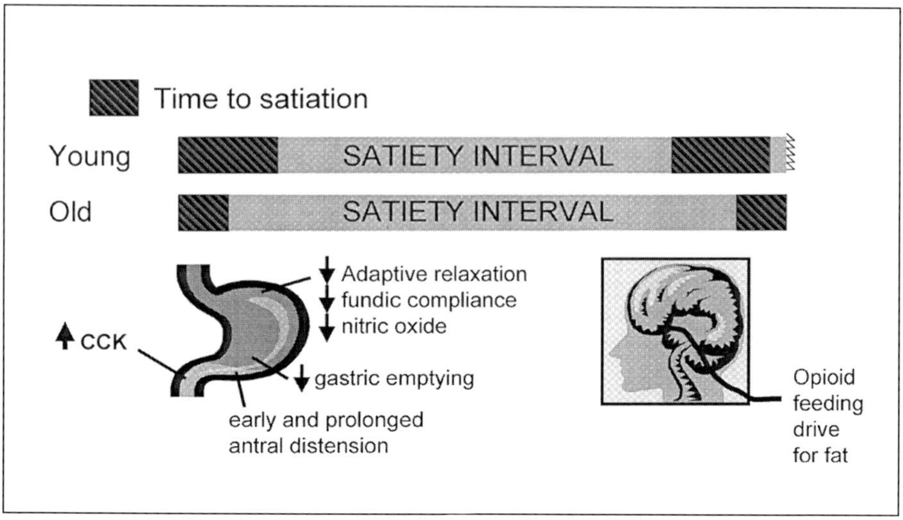

Fig. 1. Factors regulating the anorexia of aging. Effect of aging on food intake. Older persons have decreased time to satiation and prolonged satiety interval. CCK = Cholecystokinin.

experienced. Antral size is directly related to the degree of fullness experienced following a meal [5]. Infusion of liquid nutrients into the duodenum decreased the feeling of hunger in younger but not older people [6]. These findings strongly implicate the stomach in the pathogenesis of the early satiation that occurs in older people. Nitric oxide plays an important role in allowing adaptive relaxation of the fundus of the stomach. It also plays a role in increasing food intake in animals [7]. Preliminary data suggest that nitric oxide deficiency may lead to decreased fundic compliance in aging and therefore to more rapid antral filling and earlier satiation [1].

Older animals have an increased response to the satiating effect of cholecystokinin (CCK) but not to other satiating peptide hormones [8]. CCK concentrations are raised in elderly persons, particularly those with malnutrition [9]. CCK delays gastric emptying, and these studies suggest a role for CCK in the enhanced satiation seen in older people.

Older people often have impaired enjoyment of the hedonic qualities of food. The exact contribution of the changes in taste and olfaction with aging to altered food intake remains uncertain. There is a clear, universal decline in olfaction with aging [1]. The aroma of food and the release of volatile organic acids from food in the mouth are major determinants of the enjoyment of food. Decline in the different taste modes also occurs with aging, though the magnitude of change is controversial.

With aging, there is often an increase in dyspeptic symptoms. These can lead to what has been characterized as "anorexia dolorosa." The possible role of *Helicobacter pylori* and bacterial overgrowth in the small intestine in this form of anorexia remains to be determined.

Many older persons have increased circulating levels of cytokines, resulting from chronic inflammatory diseases such as arthritis. These cytokines, for example interleukin-1 and tumor necrosis factor, decrease appetite as well as increasing the prevalence of sarcopenia [10, 11]. The measurement of soluble interleukin-2 receptors appears to be a useful method to recognize this subpopulation. Severe cytokine excess will lead to decreased albumin levels, increased tryptophan entry into the brain, with an increase in serotonin and corticotropin-releasing factor (CRF) in the hypothalamus. CRF is a potent anorectic agent [12]. This syndrome has been termed pathological senile anorexia [13].

Finally, it is well documented that various central nervous system neurotransmitters are altered with aging. Many of these neurotransmitters have been involved in the modulation of food intake [14]. In particular, animal studies have suggested that the decline in opioid receptors with aging may play a pivotal role in the pathogenesis of the physiological anorexia of aging. Dynorphin, the endogenous kappa opioid receptor stimulant, plays a key role in the maintenance of fat intake. A decrease in the opioid feeding drive has been demonstrated in older animals [15]. The potential role of other neurotransmitters is deserving of more attention.

In this section we have reviewed the evidence for a physiological anorexia of aging and its multifactorial etiology (Fig. 1). In particular, it is clear that both peripheral factors, for example the rate of stomach emptying, and central nervous system factors, for example decline in the opioid feeding drive, play a role in the development of the anorexia of aging.

Causes of Malnutrition in Older Persons

There are multiple causes of protein-energy malnutrition in older persons (Table 1). These can be characterized as those due to social problems (such as poverty), psychological problems (depression), medical conditions which induce either anorexia (gallstone disease) or hypermetabolism (hyperthyroidism), drugs, and general disability (failure in the activities of daily living). It has now been shown that the most common cause of weight loss both in medical outpatient populations [16] and nursing home populations [17, 18] is depression.

We have found that physicians often fail to recognize and treat malnutrition when it occurs in older persons [16, 19]. As an aid to physicians to help to remember the causes of malnutrition in the clinical setting, we have developed the MEALS-ON-WHEELS mnemonic (Table 2) [20].

Table 1. Causes of protein-energy malnutrition

A. Social
- Poverty
- Poor food supply
- Poor eating habits

B. Psychological
- Depression
- Alcoholism
- Abuse
- Anorexia tardive/nervosa
- Late life paranoia
- Cholesterol phobia
- Globus hystericus

C. Medical causes
- (i) Anorexia
  - Gallstones
  - Dysphagia, e.g., monibasis
  - Infections
  - Cancer
  - Hypercalcemia
  - Addison's disease
  - Peptic ulcer disease
  - Gastroesophageal reflux
  - Bacterial overgrowth
- (ii) Malabsorption
  - Pancreatic disease
  - Celiac disease
- (iii) Increased metabolism
  - Hyperthyroidism
  - Pheochromocytoma
- (iv) Drugs
  - Digoxin
  - Theophylline
  - Cimetidine
  - Selective serotonin reuptake inhibitors
  - Chemotherapeutic agents
  - Neuroleptics

D. Impaired function
- Eating problems
- Inability to cook
- Inability to shop

Table 2. MEALS-ON-WHEELS mnemonic for causes of protein-energy malnutrition

M edications
E motional (depression)
A lcoholism/anorexia tardive/abuse
L ate life paranoia
S wallowing problems (dysphagia)

O ral factors
N o money (poverty)

W andering and other dementia-related problems
H yperthyroidism, hypercalcemia
E nteric problems (malabsorption)
E ating problems
L ow-salt, low-cholesterol diet
S hopping problems

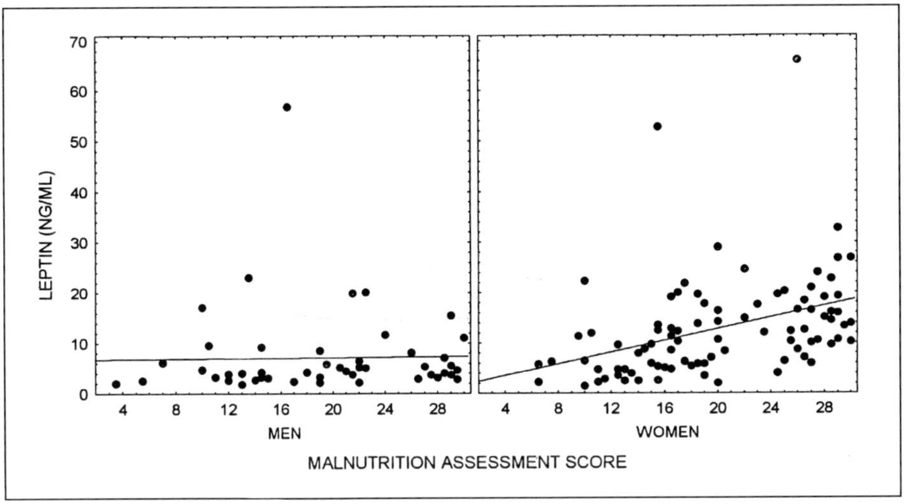

Fig. 2. Leptin levels in older men and women. Malnutrition assessment versus serum leptin in men and women.

Leptin and the Mini Nutritional Assessment

Leptin is a peptide hormone produced by adipose cells. Deficiency of leptin is responsible for the development of obesity in the genetically obese (ob/ob) mouse [21]. There is an increase in leptin concentrations at middle age, which is related to the increase in body weight and fat cell mass that occurs at that period [22]. This is then followed in females by a decline in leptin concentrations that parallels the decline in fat cell mass occurring in old age [22]. Leptin concentrations are strongly related to waist/hip ratio and the levels of the sex hormones (estradiol and testosterone). Leptin concentrations are higher in older females than males (Fig. 2). Testosterone replacement in older males with low bioavailable testosterone levels results in a decrease in leptin levels [23]. In the New Mexico Process Study of Longitudinal Aging, we found that, unlike in females, leptin concentrations increase with age in males, and this is related to the decline in testosterone [Baumgartner R, Garry PJ, Vellas B, Perry HM, and Morley JE, unpublished observations]. These data strongly argue for a role of testosterone in the regulation of leptin concentrations in males.

We have studied the relation of leptin concentrations to the MNA, using specimens collected in the Toulouse study [24]. As can be seen in Figure 3, leptin levels are highly correlated with the MNA in females, but there is no such correlation in males. The predictive factors for the MNA are given in Tables 3 and 4. An r^2 value of 0.5969 could be achieved by including age, leptin, body mass index (BMI), and albumin. A better predictive equation ($r^2 = 0.8137$) was obtained with age, leptin,

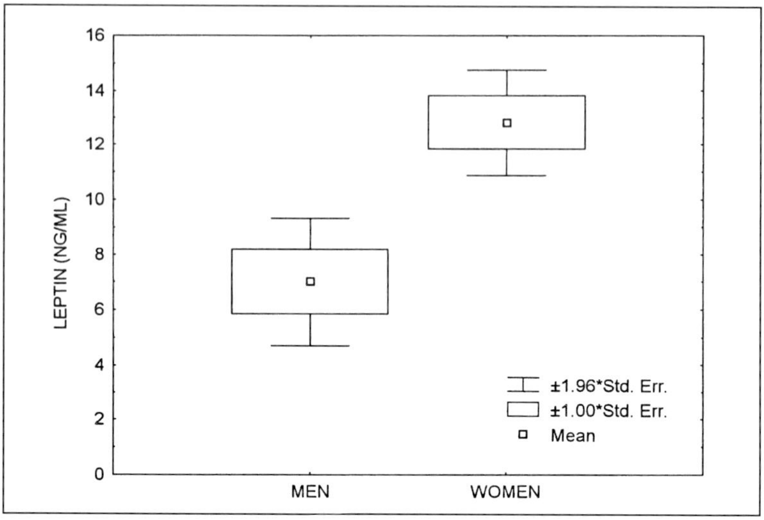

Fig. 3. Relation of leptin to the Mini Nutritional Assessment score in men and women. Serum leptin concentrations in men and women.

Table 3. Regression summary for the Mini-Nutritional Assessment ($r^2 = 0.61528541$) estimate: 3.3892

	Beta	Standard error of beta	*p* value
Age	0.280670	0.080070	0.000734
Leptin	0.182362	0.080140	0.025420
BMI	0.208090	0.080645	0.011609
Albumin	0.452926	0.080917	0.000000

BMI = Body mass index.

mini-mental status, activities of daily living, midarm muscle circumference, and ceruloplasmin. Leptin concentrations were predicted by sex, midarm circumference, albumin, and retinol binding protein ($r^2 = 0.4611$; Table 5).

The MNA and Scales in Inner City African Americans

At St. Louis University we have used a nutritional index called SCALES (Table 6) [19]. We have undertaken a large epidemiological study of aging among inner city African Americans [25]. We have previously reported that this popula-

Table 4. Regression summary for the Mini-Nutritional Assessment ($r^2 = 0.82164726$) estimate: 3.0114

	Beta	Standard error of beta	*p* value
Age	0.102933	0.041674	0.014751
Leptin	0.117580	0.038694	0.002850
MMSE	0.256797	0.060860	0.000044
ADL	0.467796	0.062408	0.000000
MAMC	0.227814	0.040354	0.000000
Ceruloplasmin	−0.098625	0.038592	0.011702

MMSE = Mini-mental status examination; ADL = activities of daily living; MAMC = midarm muscle circumference.

Table 5. Regression summary for leptin ($r^2 = 0.46113285$) estimate: 7.2991

	Beta	Standard error of beta	*p* value
Sex	0.273018	0.061156	0.000016
MAC	0.643249	0.065671	0.000000
Albumin	−0.354335	0.072764	0.000003
RBP	0.190073	0.068571	0.006305

MAC = Midarm circumference; RBP = retinol-binding protein.

tion is at high nutritional risk compared with most other elderly populations [26]. To examine the nutritional status in this group, we used our database to construct a proxy for the MNA [see Miller *et al.*, in this volume, for the methodological details]. In this chapter we examine the relation of SCALES to MNA.

The SCALES index was highly correlated with the MNA ($r^2 = -0.45730$, $p < 0.0001$, n = 101). Addition of tooth problems to the SCALES index produced a small improvement in the correlation (−0.50044), and SCALES together with illness affecting diet enhanced the correlation to −0.59150. The negative correlation is due to the fact that with the MNA the lower the score, the higher the nutritional risk, and with SCALES the higher the score, the higher the nutritional risk.

Neither SCALES nor MNA correlated significantly with BMI. Of interest was a tendency of SCALES to correlate positively with BMI, suggesting that in this population extreme overweight is a risk for the development of protein-energy malnutrition. SCALES (0.18221, $p < 0.05$) correlated with the blood urea nitrogen to creatinine ratio, whereas MNA did not (−0.14925).

Table 6. The Saint Louis University SCALES nutritional index

S	adness – geriatric depression scale of 25 or greater
C	holesterol – below 160 mg/dl
A	lbumin – below 4 g/dl
L	oss of weight – 5 pounds (2.4 kg) in 6 months
E	ating problems
S	hopping (inability to do for oneself)

1 point for each ~ maximum nutritional risk score is 6.

Table 7. Comparison of Pearson correlation coefficients for the Mini Nutritional Assessment (MNA) and SCALES end function

	SCALES	MNA
Katz ADL	0.24947 (0.0009)	–0.23608 (0.007)
Lawton IADL	0.58730 (0.0001)	–0.31172 (0.0004)
Quality of Life	–0.25443 (0.0035)	0.25987 (0.0036)
Rosow-Breslau scale	0.43763 (0.0001)	–0.40788 (0.0001)
Seven-item physical performance test	–0.35021 (0.0001)	0.21244 (0.01)
Six-meter walk (m/s)	–0.38908 (0.0001)	0.18218 (0.0952)
Time to stand five times, no arms	0.43438 (0.0001)	–0.18608 (0.0362)
Get up and go time	0.41496 (0.0001)	–0.11932 (0.1815)
Tinetti gait and balance	–0.38908 (0.0001)	0.11461 (0.1995)
Times fallen in last 3 months	0.29062 (0.0001)	–0.08568 (0.3382)
Injurious falls	0.35376 (0.0001)	–0.02956 (0.7414)
Geriatric depression scale	0.53886 (0.0001)	–0.48870 (0.0001)
Mini-mental status examination	–0.19161 (0.0113)	0.14289 (0.1090)

p values are given in parentheses.
ADL = Activities of daily living; IADL = instrumental activities of daily living.

Table 7 compares the Pearson correlation coefficients for SCALES and MNA as they relate to functional status. Both the MNA and SCALES were significantly correlated with the Katz basic activities of daily living score, the Lawton instrumental activities of daily living score, quality of life, a modified Rosow-Breslau scale of function, and the seven item physical performance test [24; Miller *et al.*, this volume, for details of these tests]. In this population, SCALES was more predictive of higher physical performance as measured by the six-meter walk, Tinetti gait and balance, time to stand eight times without using arms, and the timed get up and go test. SCALES, but not MNA, predicted falls over the last 3 months and in particular the number of injurious falls. None of these functional indices was significantly correlated with BMI.

Both SCALES and MNA were strongly correlated with the geriatric depression scale. SCALES, but not MNA, was correlated with the mini-mental state examination score. BMI was correlated with the mini-mental state score but not with the geriatric depression scale.

Overall these findings confirm the value of both the MNA and SCALES as tests of nutritional status. Both tests were strong predictors of basic functional status in this population. SCALES was a better predictor of endurance, and perhaps balance, than the MNA. The reason for this may be that the central role of albumin and cholesterol in SCALES may lead to an increased identification of diseases that would be associated with a cytokine excess, for example arthritis. In addition, SCALES identifies a number of overweight subjects with weight loss who would not be identified by the MNA but would be unlikely to be able to maintain high endurance functions. Overall, these findings confirm the role of good nutritional status in preventing functional deterioration in old age.

The fact that depression is a strong predictor of poor performance on theMNA confirms the central role of depression in the pathogenesis of protein-energy malnutrition in older persons. This finding underlines the importance of screening for depression in free living older subjects who develop weight loss. Depression is the most treatable cause of weight loss in older persons.

Summary

In this chapter we have reviewed the evidence for physiological anorexia of aging and stressed that its pathophysiology involves both central and peripheral mechanisms. Early satiation in the older person appears to involve signals predominantly arising in the stomach. The increased feeling of satiety in older persons is mainly related to changes in the central feeding drive, in particular a decrease in the opioid rewarding properties for fatty foods. Increased cytokines, secondary to inflammatory conditions which are common in old age, may further increase the anorexia seen in older persons.

Leptin, the fat hormone, is an excellent indicator of fat mass in women, in whom leptin concentrations correlate with the MNA. In men, testosterone inhibits leptin, and the fall in testosterone with age results in an increase in leptin concentrations. In males the MNA is not related to leptin concentrations.

Finally, we have examined the interrelation of two nutritional screening indices, MNA and SCALES. The two indices were well correlated and were both predictive of poor basic function. We conclude that the MNA is an excellent predictor of nutritional status. These findings suggest that malnutrition is a major predictor of frailty or the "failure to thrive" syndrome in older persons. Depression is a major cause of poor nutritional status in older persons.

References

1. Morley JE. Anorexia of aging: physiological and pathological. *Am J Clin Nutr* 1997; 66: 760–73.
2. Roberts SB, Fuss P, Heyman MB, *et al.* Control of food intake in older men. *JAMA* 1994; 272: 1601–6.
3. Wurtman JJ, Lieberman H, Tsay R, Nader T, Chew B. Calorie and nutrient intakes of elderly and young subjects measured under identical conditions. *J Gerontol* 1988; 43: B174–80.
4. Clarkston WK, Pantano MM, Morley JE, Horowitz M, Littlefield JM, Barton FR. Evidence for the anorexia of aging: gastrointestinal transit and hunger in healthy elder vs. young adults. *Am J Physiol* 1997; 41: R243–8.
5. Jones KL, Doran SM, Hveem K, *et al.* Relation between postprandial satiation and antral area in normal subjects. *Am J Clin Nutr* 1997; 66: 127–32.
6. Cook CG, Andrews JM, Jones KL, *et al.* Effects of small intestinal nutrient infusion on appetite and pyloric motility are modified by age. *Am J Physiol* 1997; 42: R755–61.
7. Morley JE, Kumar VB, Mattammal M, Villareal DT. Measurement of nitric oxide synthase and its mRNA in genetically obese (ob/ob) mice. *Life Sci* 1995; 57: 1327–31.
8. Silver AJ, Flood JF, Morley JE. Effect of gastrointestinal peptides on ingestion in young and old mice. *Peptides* 1988; 9: 221–6.
9. Berthelemy P, Bouisson M, Vellas B, *et al.* Postprandial cholecystokinin secretion in elderly with protein-energy undernutrition. *J Am Geriatr Soc* 1992; 40: 365–9.
10. Roubenoff R. Inflammatory and hormonal mediators of cachexia. *J Nutr* 1997; 127: 1014–16S.
11. Arnalich F, Hernanz A, Vazquez JJ, Amores A. Cell-mediated immune response and cytokine production in idiopathic senile anorexia. *Mech Ageing Dev* 1994; 77: 67–74.
12. Krahn DD, Gosnell BA, Levine AS, Morley JE. Behavioral effects of corticotropin-releasing factor: localization and characterization of central effects. *Brain Res* 1988; 443: 63–9.
13. Martinez M, Hernanz A, Gomez-Cerezo J, Pena JM, Vazquez JJ, Arnalich F. Alterations in plasma and cerebrospinal fluid levels of neuropeptides in idiopathic senile anorexia. *Regul Pept* 1993; 49: 109–17.
14. Morley JE. Neuropeptide regulation of appetite and weight. *Endocr Rev* 1987; 8: 256–87.
15. Gosnell BA, Levine AS, Morley JE. The effects of aging on opioid modulation of feeding in rats. *Life Sci* 1983; 32: 2793–9.
16. Wilson MMG, Vaswani S, Liu D, Morley JE, Miller DK. Prevalence and causes of undernutrition in medical outpatients. *Am J Med* 1998; 104: 56–63.
17. Morley JE, Kraenzle D. Causes of weight loss in a community nursing home. *J Am Geriatr Soc* 1994; 42: 583–5.
18. Blaum CS, Fries BE, Fiatarone MA. Factors associated with low body mass index and weight loss in nursing home residents. *J Gerontol A Biol Sci Med Sci* 1995; 50: M162–8.
19. Morley JE. Why do physicians fail to recognize and treat malnutrition in older persons? *J Am Geriatr Soc* 1991; 39: 1139–40.
20. Morley JE. Anorexia in older persons: epidemiology and optimal treatment. *Drugs Aging* 1996; 8: 134–55.
21. Friedman JM. Leptin, leptin receptors and the control of body weight. *Eur J Med Res* 1997; 2: 7–13.
22. Perry HM, Morley JE, Horowitz M, Kaiser FE, Miller DK, Witter G. Body composition and age in African American and Caucasian women: relationship to plasma leptin levels and gonadal steroids. *Metabolism* 1997; 46: 1399–1405.
23. Sih R, Morley JE, Kaiser FE, Perry HM, Patrick P, Ross C. Testosterone replacement in older hypogonadal men: a 12 month randomized controlled trial. *J Clin Endocrinol Metab* 1997; 82: 1661–7.
24. Guigoz Y, Vellas B, Garry PJ. Assessing the nutritional status of the elderly: The Mini Nutritional Assessment as part of the geriatric evaluation. *Nutr Rev* 1996; 54: S59–65.
25. Miller DK, Carter ME, Miller JP, *et al.* Inner-city older African Americans have high levels of functional disability. *J Am Geriatr Soc* 1996; 44: 1166–73.
26. Miller DK, Carter ME, Sigmund RE, *et al.* Nutritional risk in inner city dwelling African-American elderly. *J Am Geriatr Soc* 1996; 44: 959–62.

Discussion

Unidentified participant: It looks as though the correlation between MNA and the SCALES was quite good, but they diverged a lot for certain predictors. Do you have an explanation for this?

Dr. Morley: I think the basic difference between MNA and SCALES is the laboratory tests. Otherwise they are very similar. The screening approach to someone who is malnourished should be to do the simplest screening test, which would be the MNA, and if there appears to be malnutrition, to follow this up with at least an albumin and a cholesterol determination. This will identify people who are malnourished but with less weight loss – in other words those who are really developing kwashiorkor. I think the SCALES are more useful for the kwashiorkor rather than the marasmic type of picture. Most older people appear marasmic, but the subset with a kwashiorkor-like picture do worse. The other possibility is that SCALES also reflect cytokine activity, because as we know the cytokines – particularly tumor necrosis factor and interleukin-1 and 2 – will cause a reduction in albumin and cholesterol. So you may be getting a mixed picture with SCALES, one that particularly identifies frailty because these are people who also have other processes going on that interfere with muscle strength.

Unidentified participant: It is surprising that there is such a strong correlation between the MNA and albumin.

Dr. Morley: The strongest correlations with the MNA have been over periods of time or in larger populations. The MNA seems to be good at reflecting early malnutrition, while the SCALES will pick up later more full-blown nutritional disease. Over time, the MNA predicts albumin very well in large populations, because the MNA identifies the ill malnourished person. But the MNA also picks up a group that is at risk a little earlier than the SCALES – that is, a healthier population more likely to develop problems in the future if you don't interfere. That makes the MNA a very good test in this setting.

Dr. Schiffrin: Does this diminution of nitric oxide synthase that you showed in the stomach occur in the muscle layer, and is this local diminution also general in the rest of the body? Could it, for example, explain hypertension?

Dr. Morley: In the stomach, we measured the whole stomach layer, but it was mainly smooth muscle, not endothelium that we were measuring. As to the second part of your question, this is a fascinating area, and I'm going to give you my best guess. We have looked at NOS in monocytes and have shown that it increases with age, unlike in endothelium and in the fundus of the stomach. Therefore there is more circulating nitric oxide as we get older. I think this increase in circulating nitric oxide downregulates the changes that we are seeing in the endothelium and in the stomach. So the monocyte appears to be driving the other changes. It seems likely that it does play a major role in the development of hypertension, and we also have some data suggesting that tumor necrosis factor α is involved in the production of diabetes in older people and the hyperglycemia of aging, and that insulin resistance is dependent on nitric oxide. We think the syndrome X, which is well described in middle aged and older people, is due to this excess production of nitric oxide.

Dr. Schiffrin: You emphasize that monocytes are activated in the elderly. Do you mean in general, no matter what the nutritional state?

Dr. Morley: I can't tell you whether or not it is related to nutrition; we are looking at that at the moment. Maybe one of the questions that would be worthwhile asking, particularly in relation to the use of MNA, is whether you cause changes in the nitric oxide levels by nutritional rehabilitation.

Mini Nutritional Assessment (MNA): Research and Practice in the Elderly:
B. Vellas; P.J. Garry; Y. Guigoz (eds),
Nestlé Nutrition Workshop Series Clinical & Performance Programme, Vol. 1, pp. 79–86,
Nestec Ltd.; Vevey/S. Karger AG, Basel, © 1999.

Associations among the Mini Nutritional Assessment Instrument, Dehydration, and Functional Status among Older African Americans in St. Louis, Mo., USA

Douglas K. Miller, Horace M. Perry III and John E. Morley

Division of Geriatric Medicine, St. Louis University Health Sciences Center; Geriatric Research, Education, and Clinical Center, St. Louis Veterans Affairs Medical Center; St. Louis, Mo., USA

Nutritional integrity is clearly essential for health in older persons [1], and the Mini Nutritional Assessment (MNA) instrument has been shown to be an effective measure of risk of nutritional failure in older individuals [2]. We have previously demonstrated that dehydration is also associated with adverse functional outcomes in older persons [3], and data from other investigators support this conclusion as well [4–6]. However, it is unclear to what extent measures of nutritional status, and specifically the MNA, are associated with dehydration and its adverse functional correlates. In this study, we investigated those relations among a group of 138 older African Americans from inner city St. Louis, Mo., USA.

Methods

Participants

The basic study design has been described previously in detail [7, 8]. In brief, a sample frame of all persons aged 70 years and older living in the catchment area was developed using lists from the Health Care Finance Administration's Medicare enrollment eligibility file, and those persons who either lived in a nursing home or identified themselves as white (2%) were removed. Six hundred and twelve persons were selected at random from the sample frame and approached for participation, of whom 416 (68%) were recruited and interviewed. An addi-

Table 1. Comparison of the modified Mini-Nutritional Assessment in St. Louis PFUAA study to published version*

No.	Item	Comment	Fidelity
1	Body mass index	Identical	High
2	Mid-arm circumference	Identical	High
3	Calf circumference	(Not available)	(No data)
4	Weight loss	Identical	High
5	Independent at home	No institutionalized subjects	Moderate
6	>3 prescription drugs per day	Identical	High
7	Stress or acute disease	"Illness or condition changed my eating"	Moderate
8	Mobility	Identical	High
9	Neuropsychological problems	MMSE and GDS, usual cutpoints	High
10	Pressure sores or skin ulcers	By observation	High
11	Number of meals per day	1 (0 pts) vs ≥2 (1.5 pts) meals per day	Moderate
12	Protein intake	Milk ≥5/wk (1 pt); otherwise (0.5 pt)	Fair to poor
13	Fruits and vegetables	One or more of each = 1 point	Moderate
14	Appetite or oral difficulties	Self-rate appetite (poor = 0, fair = 1, rest = 2)	Moderate
15	Fluid intake	(Not available)	(No data)
16	Feeding dependence	Need assistance = 0, self-feed = 2	Moderate
17	Self-rated nutrition	DETERMINE scale, published cutpoints	Moderate
18	Self-rated health	Fair or poor = 0, good = 1, > good = 2	Moderate

Max. score = 27.5.
* Guigoz Y, *et al.* [2].

tional 230 subjects were recruited from senior citizen apartments and from programs associated with a community service organization that worked in the catchment area. From these participants, 168 persons were recruited into a physical evaluation focused on their strength, balance, body habitus, and nutritional status. Blood was obtained from 174 subjects for testing; 134 of these subjects had received strength and balance evaluation, and 40 had not. These 134 subjects constitute the study group for the current investigation.

Approval was obtained from the St. Louis University (SLU) Health Sciences Center's Institutional Review Board for all research procedures. Informed consent was obtained from all recruited participants in conformance with the assurance given by SLU to the Department of Health and Human Services to protect the rights of human subjects.

Measurements

Data were available to measure 16 of the 18 items comprising the MNA (Table 1). It should be noted that data regarding calf circumference and fluid intake were not available in the St. Louis data set and are therefore not included in the modified MNA. The other items in the modified MNA showed good to excellent agreement with the comparable items in the published version of the MNA [2]. Our version of the MNA had a maximum of 27.5 points compared with a maxi-

Table 2. MNA levels in St. Louis PFUAA study

MNA category (criteria)	Prevalence
Well nourished (≥ 22)	59.8%
At risk malnutrition (15.5–21.5)	38.6%
Malnutrition (≤ 15)	1.6%

mum of 30 points in the published version. Cutoff points for nutritional status were adjusted for the difference in maximum points as follows: 22 or above, well-nourished; 15.5 to 21.5, at risk of malnutrition; less than 15.5, frank malnutrition (Table 2).

Creatinine (Cr), blood urea nitrogen (BUN), and the ratio of BUN to Cr (BUN/Cr) were measured by a reliable commercial laboratory. BUN/Cr was used as the indicator of dehydration, and the laboratory's published upper limit of normal of 18 was accepted as the highest normal value for the BUN/Cr.

All frailty-dependent variables were obtained without knowledge of the laboratory tests. Dependent variables based on the interview included the following. Basic activities of daily living (ADL) were measured using the six-item Katz scale [9], and intermediate activities of daily living (IADL) were measured using the eight-item Lawton & Brody scale [10]; both scales were scored as the number of items requiring personal assistance. The modification of the Rosow-Breslau scale by Guralnik *et al.* [11] was employed to measure higher ADL functioning and was scored from 0 to 3 for the inability (a) to walk up and down a full flight of stairs, (b) to walk half a mile (0.8 km), or (c) to do heavy work around the house without assistance. Interviewers also obtained the geriatric depression scale (GDS) [12] and a structured form [13] of the mini-mental state examination (MMSE) [14].

Frailty-dependent variables based on the strength and balance examination included the following. Balance was evaluated using the timed one-leg stand with eyes open (as described and validated by Bohannon *et al.* [15]), and a standing balance scale developed by Guralnik *et al.* [16] (range 0–4 from worst to best). Ability to perform walking tasks was measured using the timed "Up and Go" test of Podsiadlo & Richardson [17]; in this test the subject arises from a firm chair, walks 3 m, turns around, returns to the chair, and sits down again as quickly as possible. Overall physical capabilities were measured with the seven item physical performance test (PPT-7) of Reuben & Siu [18]. This test involves lifting a moderately heavy book to shoulder height, writing a sentence, simulated eating using beans and a tin can, donning/doffing a jacket, picking a penny off the floor, turning 360 degrees while standing, and walking at preferred gait speed. During the physical assessment, subjects were also questioned regarding their overall subjective quality of life, using the QL index uniscale developed and validated by Spitzer *et al.* [19].

Each of the dependent variables was coded such that a lower number represented greater frailty. For the MMSE, Guralnik stance, PPT-7, and quality-of-life variables, this required reversing the direction of the originally described measure. For correlations with the frailty-dependent variables, the MNA was recoded so that a higher number represented worse nutritional status, to improve cross comparisons with the BUN/Cr.

Comparison of Participants and Non-Participants

As reported previously [3], those having blood tests were in slightly better health than subjects not having such tests. They reported somewhat fewer basic ADL dependencies, fewer IADL dependencies, better Rosow-Breslau functioning, and higher MMSE. However, there were no significant differences in age, sex, GDS score, one-leg stand time, Guralnik stance performance, "Up and Go" time, or quality of life.

Statistical Analysis

The Pearson product moment correlation was used to test the relation between two continuous variables, and Student's *t* test was used to test differences in a continuous variable between two groups (for example, well-nourished *versus* at risk or malnourished on the MNA). As in the previous study [3], the one-leg stand time was log-normal transformed to improve the distribution of residuals.

To evaluate whether the MNA and BUN/Cr both contributed explained variance to the dependent variables or were significantly colinear in their explanatory contribution, multiple linear regression was used to evaluate the effect of one variable while controlling for the other. Analyses involving the one leg timed stand again used the log-normal transformed value.

Results

Study Group

Salient characteristics of the study sample have been published previously [3, 7] and will be reviewed only briefly here. Average age was 79.7 years, and 68% were female. Twenty-seven percent indicated that they were in fair or poor health. Subjects averaged 1.06 IADL dependencies, and very few met criteria for depression or dementia. Physical measures were systematically worse than in relevant comparison groups [7]. In this sample, using the modified criteria above, 6 of 10 subjects were well-nourished, nearly 4 of 10 were at risk of malnutrition, and only 1.6% were actually malnourished (Table 2).

MNA and Dehydration

Poor nutritional status, as measured by the modified MNA, was weakly and nonsignificantly associated with the BUN/Cr ratio. The correlation between the

Table 3. MNA versus dehydration, as measured by BUN/Cr, in the St. Louis PFUAA study (by t test)

MNA category	BUN/Cr
Well-nourished	13.2 (SD 4.1)
At risk or malnourished	14.0 (SD 3.2)
	$p = 0.267$

BUN = Blood urea nitrogen; Cr = serum creatinine.

Table 4. Bivariable analyses of MNA and dehydration versus functional and quality of life measures in St. Louis PFUAA study

Item	Correlation (p value)	
	MNA	BUN/Cr
Katz basic ADL	0.236 (0.008)	0.179 (0.018)[+]
Lawton IADL	0.312 (0.0004)	0.315 (0.0001)[+]
Rosow-Breslau	0.408 (0.0001)	0.274 (0.0002)[+]
GDS	0.489 (0.0001)	0.203 (0.008)[+]
MMSE	0.143 (0.109)	0.045 (0.556)
One-leg stand time	0.038 (0.673)	0.274 (0.002)[+]*
Guralnik stance	0.158 (0.084)	0.325 (0.0002)[+]*
Timed "Up & Go"	0.119 (0.182)	0.260 (0.002)[+]
PPT-7	0.212 (0.017)	0.260 (0.002)[+]
QOL	0.260 (0.004)	0.215 (0.014)[+]

QOL = Quality of life. See Methods section for other abbreviations.

[+] Still significant after controlling for creatinine and sodium [3].

* Still significant after controlling for BUN as well as creatinine and sodium [3].

two factors, treated as continuous variables, was 0.15 ($p = 0.14$), and the t test showed a nonsignificant trend (Table 3).

Among the functional outcome variables, the MNA was associated with basic and IADL dependencies, Rosow-Breslau scale, GDS, PPT-7, and quality of life (Table 4). On the other hand, the MNA was not associated with one-leg stand time, Guralnik stance, or "Up and Go" time, while the BUN/Cr was strongly associated with all three. When compared with the bivariable analyses in Table 4, the multivariable results indicated moderate shared explanatory variance between the MNA and BUN/Cr for the Katz basic ADL and PPT-7; small shared explanatory variance for Lawton IADLs and quality of life; and minimal to no shared variance for Rosow-Breslau, GDS, one-leg stand time, Guralnik stance performance, and timed "Up and Go" (Table 5).

Table 5. Multivariable analyses of MNA and dehydration versus functional and quality of life measures in St. Louis PFUAA study

Item	Standardized beta (*p* value)	
	MNA	BUN/Cr
Katz basic ADL	0.120 (0.230)	0.201 (0.045)
Lawton IADL	0.253 (0.009)	0.243 (0.012)
Rosow-Breslau	0.341 (0.0003)	0.279 (0.0025)
GDS	0.460 (0.0001)	0.183 (0.038)
MMSE	0.111 (0.274)	0.045 (0.660)
One-leg stand time	0.042 (0.673)	0.252 (0.013)
Guralnik stance	0.170 (0.081)	0.330 (0.001)
Timed "Up & Go"	0.094 (0.336)	0.265 (0.008)
PPT-7	0.143 (0.148)	0.197 (0.048
QOL	0.194 (0.048)	0.259 (0.009)

Abbreviations as noted in Table 4. All analyses control one independent variable (e.g., MNA) for the effect of the other (e.g., BUN/Cr).

Conclusion

The MNA has been shown to be associated with important functional outcomes. We have previously demonstrated associations between obesity and fear of falling and between increased abdomen-to-hip ratio and greater ADL dependencies and worse performance on the one-leg stand time and PPT-7 [20]. We have also shown strong associations between dehydration and adverse functional outcomes [3]. Thus both proper nutrition and hydration status appear important for maintaining health and functioning in older persons.

However, the impacts of nutritional status (at least as measured by this modified version of the MNA) and dehydration on functional outcomes appear to operate through separate mechanisms. That is, although the MNA reflects nutritional status, it does not appear to reflect hydration status particularly well. This conclusion is supported by the lack of direct association between the two variables, the different impacts on functional outcomes in the bivariable analyses, and the minimal colinearity in the multivariable analyses. Whether nutritional status and dehydration status have by nature separate pathophysiological mechanisms, or whether the MNA is not strongly associated with dehydration while other measures of nutritional status reflect dehydration status better will require additional investigation. Ultimately, however, it may be necessary to separate the measurement of nutritional and hydration status. In this case, new and more direct measures of hydration status and risk of dehydration will have to be designed and validated.

Other possible explanations for the low level of association between the MNA and dehydration in our study are the modifications in the MNA required in our dataset and the inner city African American population comprising our study sample. Our measurement of dehydration is quite standard and has been found previously to show the expected associations with functional outcomes [3], so an invalid measurement of dehydration appears an unlikely explanation for the limited association. It remains to be seen whether some of the findings relate to the specific demographic characteristics of our sample or the conclusions are stable across different race, ethnic, and age groups. Also the processes involved in selecting the 138 participants for this study from the 646 total interviewed sample might explain some of the findings. Although we have shown that selection biases, as far as we could measure them, were relatively few and mild, they may have produced some of the findings.

In summary, both nutritional status and dehydration status are important for full health for older persons. However, the MNA as one measure of nutritional status does not reflect hydration status particularly well. This may be because of measurement issues peculiar to this study, but it is more likely that nutritional status and hydration status need to be measured separately.

Acknowledgment

Supported by Grant No. 5 RO1 AG10436 from the National Institute on Aging's Minority Physical Frailty program.

References

1. Morley JE. Anorexia of aging: physiologic and pathologic. *Am J Clin Nutr* 1997; 66: 760–73.
2. Guigoz Y, Vellas B, Garry PJ. Mini Nutritional Assessment: a practical assessment tool for grading the nutritional state of elderly patients. *Facts Res Gerontol* 1994; (suppl 2): 15–59.
3. Miller DK, Perry HM, Morley JE. Relationship of dehydration and chronic renal insufficiency with function and cognitive status in older US blacks. *Facts Res Gerontol* 1998; (Special issue): 149–59.
4. Lavizzo-Mourey R, Johnson J, Stolley P. Risk factors for dehydration among elderly nursing home residents. *J Am Geriatr Soc* 1988; 36: 213–18.
5. Vital and Health Statistics from the Centers for Disease Control and Prevention/National Center for Health Statistics. *Detailed Diagnoses and Procedures, National Hospital Discharge Survey 1991.* Washington, DC: US Department of Health and Human Services, 1994.
6. Warren JL, Bacon WE, Harris T, McBean AM, Foley DJ, Phillips C. The burden and outcomes associated with dehydration among US elderly, 1991. *Am J Public Health* 1994; 84: 1265–9.
7. Miller DK, Carter ME, Miller JP, *et al.* Inner-city older blacks have high levels of functional disability. *J Am Geriatr Soc* 1996; 44: 1166–73.
8. Miller DK, Carter ME, Sigmund RH, *et al.* Nutritional risk in inner-city-dwelling older black Americans. *J Am Geriatr Soc* 1996; 44: 959–62.
9. Katz S, Ford AB, Moskowitz RW, Jackson BA, Jaffe MW. Studies of illness in the aged. The index of ADL: a standardized measure of biological and psychosocial function. *JAMA* 1963; 185: 914–19.
10. Lawton MP, Brody EM. Assessment of older people: self-maintaining and instrumental activities of daily living. *Gerontologist* 1969; 9: 179–86.
11. Guralnik JM, LaCroix AZ, Branch LG, Kasl SV, Wallace RB. Morbidity and disability in older persons in the years prior to death. *Am J Public Health* 1991; 81: 443–7.

12. Yesavage JA, Brink TL, Rose TL, *et al.* Development and validation of a geriatric depression screening scale: a preliminary report. *J Psychiatr Res* 1982–3; 17: 37–49.
13. Molloy DW, Alemayehu E, Roberts R. Reliability of a standardized Mini-Mental State Examination compared with the traditional Mini-Mental State Examination. *Am J Psychiatry* 1991; 148: 102–5.
14. Folstein MF, Folstein SE, McHugh PR. "Mini-mental state." A practical method for grading the cognitive state of patients for the clinician. *J Psychiatr Res* 1975; 12: 189–98.
15. Bohannon RW, Larkin PA, Cook AC, Gear J, Singer J. Decrease in time balance test scores with aging. *Phys Ther* 1984; 64: 1067–70.
16. Guralnik JM, Simonsick EM, Ferrucci L, *et al.* A short physical performance battery assessing lower extremity function: association with self-reported disability and prediction of mortality and nursing home admission. *J Gerontol* 1994; 49: M85–94.
17. Podsiadlo D, Richardson S. The timed "Up & Go": a test of basic functional mobility for frail elderly persons. *J Am Geriatr Soc* 1991; 39: 142–8.
18. Reuben DB, Siu AL. An objective measure of physical function of elderly outpatients: the physical performance test. *J Am Geriatr Soc* 1990; 38: 1105–12.
19. Spitzer WO, Dobson AJ, Hall J, *et al.* Measuring the quality of life of cancer patients: a concise QL-index for use by physicians. *J Chron Dis* 1981; 34: 585–97.
20. Miller DK, Lantigua R, Miles TP. Relationship between malnutrition and physical frailty in three minority populations (abstract). *Gerontologist* 1995; 35 (special issue 1, Oct): 158–9.

Discussion

Unidentified participant: Do you expect to have stronger correlation with hydration if you have more people in the malnourished range, or do you think that the effects of hydration and malnutrition operate by quite different mechanisms?

Dr. Miller: My guess is that we need to look at them as two different constructs. Since most adverse events in older people have multiple components, it's not surprising that there will be some overlap between nutrition and hydration, but with such a low correlation I think we need to look for something that really defines those patients who are at risk of dehydration. This is an area for more research.

Dr. Chumlea: With your African American population, to what extent is the dehydration effect that you're seeing influenced by the classical high salt content of the African American diet?

Dr. Miller: We don't have much on the nutritional content of their diet. We do know that about a third of them were on diuretics, and about the same proportion reported having reduced the salt in their diet, though they still eat a lot of pork and other high salt foods. About 35% were born and raised in St. Louis, but almost all the rest came from southern states where the diet is very high in salt. Although our data may be culturally limited there could be more general implications.

Dr. Ferry: Don't you think that there are two phenomena here? Malnutrition is a long process and dehydration can be a short and dangerous one. It seems improbable that one test would be applicable to two such different conditions. I don't believe MNA is likely to be a good tool for dehydration.

Dr. Miller: We can probably do a better job of defining the people who are at risk for dehydration, and once we can be more certain of identifying the risk factors for dehydration we will then be in a better position to see if the two conditions can be recognized by a single test. But I agree, the chances are that it will need to be treated as a separate construct.

Dr. Morley: I totally agree. It is a good thing that the MNA does not tap into dehydration; if it did, the test would emerge as much more global and less specific. I believe the MNA is very specific for nutritional status. There are more and more data suggesting that it is a nutritional tool and that poor nutrition then taps into frailty and other things. Also, from the point of view of population limitations, it looks as though there is not a major ethnic difference in MNA results.

Mini Nutritional Assessment (MNA): Research and Practice in the Elderly:
B. Vellas; P.J. Garry; Y. Guigoz (eds),
Nestlé Nutrition Workshop Series Clinical & Performance Programme, Vol. 1, pp. 87–92,
Nestec Ltd.; Vevey/S. Karger AG, Basel, © 1999.

Mini Nutritional Assessment and Alzheimer Patients

F. Nourhashemi[a], S. Guyonnet[a], P.J. Ousset[a], V. Kostek, S. Lauque, W.C. Chumlea[b], B. Vellas[a], and J.L. Albarède[b]

[a] *Alzheimer Special Unit, Department of Internal Medicine and Clinical Gerontology, Toulouse University Hospital, Toulouse, France;* [b] *Wright State University, School of Medicine, Dayton, Ohio, USA*

Weight loss, behavioral problems, and food disorders are common in patients with Alzheimer disease. Recently, White *et al.* [1] found that weight loss was present in 36% of Alzheimer disease patients compared with 18% in controls. These changes in weight occur not only in patients with severe dementia, but may precede dementia. Barrett-Connor *et al.* [2] followed 134 older men and 165 women for 20 years in a longitudinal study on aging, and found weight loss before the onset of Alzheimer disease. Many attempts have been made in the past few years to understand this weight loss in Alzheimer patients. Barrett-Connor and colleagues found no evidence of a higher resting metabolic rate in non-institutionalized Alzheimer patients [3]. More recently, Poehlman *et al.* [4] did not find any differences in daily energy expenditure in Alzheimer patients compared with healthy controls. However, Grundman *et al.* [5] found that low body weight in Alzheimer disease is associated with mesial temporal cortical atrophy.

The ELSA Study

The ELSA study is a longitudinal study on a population of Alzheimer patients. Age at entry was 74.6 ± 7.0 years; 32.5% of the subjects were men and 67.5% women; 23% lived alone, 71% with their family, and 6% were in institutions. The mean mini-mental state (MMSE) assessment score at entry was 14.9 ± 6, and none of the patients had more than two abnormalities at the activities of daily living (ADL) scale. The mean Mini Nutritional Assessment (MNA) score was 24

Table 1. Weight loss in Alzheimer disease: the ELSA study

	Weight loss (>4%)			
	Jo		J12	
	No (n = 42)	Yes (n = 34)	No (n = 42)	Yes (n = 34)
MMSE	16.2±6	13.4±7.1*	13.5±8.9	9.9±6.7*
MNA	24±2.3	24.7±2	23.8±12.3	22.4±3.6*
Weight (kg)	61.4±13	62.5±13	62.5±14.8	57±14.5**
Energy intake (kcal)	2,013±652	1,909±473	1,891±694	1,772±413
C-Reactive protein (mg %)	4.4±4.3	4.1±3.7	5.8±6.4	8.1±17
Serum albumin (g/l)	44.9±4	43.3±4.6	43±5	44±5.1

MMSE = Mini mental state examination score; MNA = Mini Nutritional Assessment score.

* $p < 0.05$.

** $p < 0.01$.

± 2.3; 57% had an MNA of >23.5, 37% between 17 and 23.5, and 6% of <17. The mean energy intake in this population was 2,013 ± 652 kcal; however, 25% had an energy intake of <1,500 kcal/day. None of these people had inflammatory disease, and the mean plasma C-reactive protein concentration was 4.4 ± 4.3 mg/dl.

Over a one-year period of follow-up, we found a clinically significant weight loss (>4%; [6] in 44.2% of these Alzheimer patients; 13% had a weight loss of >10%. As can be seen in Tables 1 and 2, weight loss was related to a significant decrease in the MNA score over a one-year period, from 24.7 ± 2 to 22.4 ± 3.6 ($p < 0.05$) in those who experienced a weight lost of >4%, and from 23.8 ± 7 to 20.9 ± 3.5 ($p < 0.05$) for those who experienced a weight lost of >10%.

However, we did not find any change in serum albumin in these patients. It seems that the MNA (but not the serum albumin) is useful in following nutritional status in these Alzheimer patients. We also found that weight changes were correlated with the Zaritt score, which classifies the burden of the disease on the family [7]. Recently, Fredman & Daly [8] found that weight change is an indicator of caregiver stress in Alzheimer patients. Like other teams, we found no difference in energy expenditure in Alzheimer patients who experienced weight loss compared with those who did not [9, 10]. It also seems that when we take the burden on the family into consideration, the severity of dementia alone is not related to the MNA score. For example, we found an MNA score of 21.2 ± 4.0 in patients with an MMSE score of <5 compared with 23.6 ± 2.2 in those with a score of >5. However, the MNA appears to be related to eating behavior in Alzheimer patients

Table 2. Weight loss in Alzheimer disease: the ELSA study

	Weight loss (>10%)			
	Jo		J12	
	No (n = 42)	Yes (n = 10)	No (n = 42)	Yes (n = 10)
MMSE	16.2±6	12.7±6*	13.5±8.9	8.7±6.5*
MNA	24±2.3	23.8±7	23.8±12.3	20.9±3.5*
Weight (kg)	61.4±13	59.3±14	62.5±14.8	51±12.9**
Energy intake (kcal)	2,013±652	1,941±482	1,891±694	1,565±335
C-Reactive protein (mg %)	4.4±4.3	5.8±6.5	5.8±6.4	6.9±7
Serum albumin (g/l)	44.9±4	40.1±5	43±5	44±4.2

MMSE = Mini mental state examination score; MNA = Mini Nutritional Assessment score.

* $p<0.05$.

** $p<0.01$.

[11]. We found that of those with an MMSE score of <10, 22.9% needed to be fed intermittently, 8.8% puckered their lips preventing food entry, 11.8% needed coaxing or would not eat, 14.7% use fingers instead of utensils, and 2.9% accepted only liquid food.

MNA Score in Alzheimer Disease Inpatients

Special care units appear to be beneficial for Alzheimer disease patients. Two years ago, we started an EC-funded study on Alzheimer disease special care units in Europe: a case-control study on quality of life for patients and family. Involved in this study are special care units in nursing homes in Italy (Brescia) and Sweden (Karolinska Institute), while in France, we elected to study the Toulouse acute care unit for Alzheimer patients [12–15], one of the first acute care units for Alzheimer patients in Europe. Alzheimer patients are admitted to this unit from their home, from nursing homes, or from the hospital emergency department for complications related or unrelated to Alzheimer disease. We provide medical management for Alzheimer patients, while patients with other conditions only have an assessment of cognitive function.

Table 3 summarizes our data on the first 118 Alzheimer disease patients in 1996; 59% were women, mean age 78.6 ± 8.3 years, 70% came from home, and 20% from nursing homes. The mean MNA score was 19.6 ± 4.9, lower than in Alzheimer patients living in the community as determined in the ELSA study,

Table 3. ELSA: Description of the population (n = 88)

Age at entry (years)		74.6 ± 7.0
Sex	Men	32.5%
	Women	67.5%
Living conditions	Alone	23%
	With family	71%
	Institution	6%
MMS		14.9 ± 6
GDS	3	17%
	4	40%
	5	33%
	6	10%
MNA		24 ± 2.3
ADL		<2 abnormalities

MMS = Mini mental state examination score; GDS = geriatric depression scale; MNA = Mini Nutritional Assessment score; ADL = activities daily living score.

and 32% had food intakes lower than two thirds of the RDA. Other studies have found that the nutritional status of Alzheimer disease patients is better in special care units than in regular care facilities [14]. Cause of death in Alzheimer disease patients is mainly bronchopneumonia (64%) [16]. We think that if we can improve nutritional status and immunologic function in such patients, we should be able to decrease the risk of such infections.

Conclusions

In conclusion, weight loss and malnutrition are frequent in Alzheimer patients. The MNA is easy to use and useful in these patients, though some of the questions need to be answered by the caregiver. MNA (but not albumin) is correlated with weight loss in Alzheimer patients. The severity of dementia is a risk factor for malnutrition, but in those living at home, MNA score and MMSE are not correlated. It seems possible to prevent malnutrition and weight loss in many Alzheimer patients. For these reasons, we have started a European-funded program on nutrition health promotion and Alzheimer disease for health professionals and caregivers. This program will be translated into 11 languages and disseminated throughout Europe.

References

1. White H, Pieper C, Schmader K, Fillenbaum G. Weight change in Alzheimer's disease. *J Am Geriatr Soc* 1996; 44: 265–72.
2. Barrett-Connor E, Edelstein SL, Corey-Bloom J, Wiederholt WC. Weight loss precedes dementia in community-dwelling older adults. *J Am Geriatr Soc* 1996; 44: 1147–52.
3. Barrett-Connor E, Donaldson KE, Carpenter WH, *et al.* No evidence for higher resting metabolic rate in noninstitutionalized Alzheimer's disease patients. *J Am Geriatr Soc* 1996; 44: 1232–4.
4. Poehlman ET, Toth MJ, Goran MI, Carpenter WH, Newhouse P, Rosen CJ. Daily energy expenditure in free-living non-institutionalized Alzheimer's patients: a doubly labeled water study. *Neurology* 1997; 48: 997–1002.
5. Grundman M, Corey-Bloom J, Jernigan T, Archibald S, Thal LJ. Loss of body weight in Alzheimer's disease is associated with mesial temporal cortex atrophy. *Neurology* 1996; 46: 1585–91.
6. Wallace JI, Schwartz RS, LaCroix AZ, Uhlmann RF, Pearlman RA. Involuntary weight loss in older outpatients: incidence and clinical significance. *J Am Geriatr Soc* 1995; 43: 329–37.
7. Zarit SH, Todd PA, Zarit JM. Families under stress: interventions for caregivers of senile dementia patients. *Psychotherapy* 1982; 19: 461–71.
8. Fredman L, Daly MP. Weight change: an indicator of caregiver stress. *J Aging Health* 1997; 9: 43–69.
9. Guyonnet S, Nourhashemi F, Andrieu S, *et al.* A prospective study of changes in the nutritional status of Alzheimer's patients. *Arch Gerontol Geriatr* 1998; suppl 6: 255–62.
10. Reves G, Guyonnet S, Nourhashemi F, Vellas B. Weight loss in Alzheimer's disease and resting energy expenditure (REE), a preliminary report. *J Am Geriatr Soc* (in press)
11. Blandford G, Mulvihill M, Taylor B. Assessing abnormal feeding behavior in dementia: a taxonomy and initial findings. In: *Research in practice in Alzheimer's disease.* New York: Springer, 1998: 47–64.
12. Nourhashemi F, Vellas B, *et al.* Medical management and non-cognitive aspects of Alzheimer's disease. In: *Research in practice in Alzheimer's disease.* New York: Springer, 1998: 233–248.
13. Vellas BJ, Nourhashemi F, Ousset PJ, Albarede JL. Alzheimer's disease and geriatric medicine. *Korean J Gerontol* 1997; 7: 63–70.
14. Nourhashemi F, Vellas B, Albarede JL. Special care acute unit for Alzheimer's patients. In: Geriatrics department and facilities. *Facts Res Intervent Geriatr* 1998 (in press).
15. Nourhashemi F, Ousset PJ, Vellas B. Acute inhospital Alzheimer units are investigated in Europe. *J Am Geriatr Soc* 1997; 45: 861–2.
16. Burns A, Jacoby R, Luthert P, Levy R. Cause of death in Alzheimer's disease. *Age Ageing* 1990; 19: 341–4.

Discussion

Dr. Chumlea: In your work where the MNA was done in Alzheimer patients, obviously the answers to the MNA were from a caregiver?

Dr. Vellas: For some of the questions.

Dr. Chumlea: That's fine. My recommendation though is that if you are going to collect MNA questions about a patient from the caregiver, then one should also administer the MNA independently to the caregiver: if the caregiver had an MNA of, say 23, there might be a relation between the nutrition of the caregiver and the nutrition of the patient. So it might be beneficial – in some of those instances at least – to look at those relations.

Dr. Vellas: That's true, especially because we know that Alzheimer disease is a disease of the family. For many aspects of the disease – for example depression or quality of life – we have found that the problems of the patient are shared by the caregiver. Maybe it is the same with nutrition.

To answer the question about subjective assessment, what we need to do is to teach physicians and others how to use MNA. If elderly people cannot respond to the subjective questions, health professionals need to decide the answer on the basis of their own impressions – that's the way it works, the MNA is validated like that. Many of the problems in using the MNA are caused by lack of education in its use.

Dr. Morley: When you looked at your Alzheimer patients, did you look to see how many of those at home were wanderers, and how that affected both their nutritional status and the question of caregiver abuse? We find two major reasons for weight loss in Alzheimer patients: one is anorexia, but the other is a smaller group of people who wander all the time – they just do not stop going. Those people use a lot of energy, but they are also very burdensome to the caregiver and this may be part of the correlation with the caregiver burden that you see.

Dr. Vellas: In our population, we have people with mild to moderate dementia, and we don't have any with wandering problems. The only significant correlation was with the burden on the family.

Dr. Arnaud-Battandier: If you had to develop a nutritional program, what would you recommend?

Dr. Vellas: Our hypothesis is that weight loss in Alzheimer patients is mostly a consequence of a poor intake at some point in the disease. For example, at the onset of the disease, an elderly person living alone will often purchase and prepare less food. If we can detect malnutrition at this time, for example by using the MNA, and give help to the patient, our hypothesis is that we could decrease weight loss in this population.

Dr. Rubenstein: As a general statement, both cancer patients and Alzheimer patients are ideal patients for nutritional screening, and nutritional intervention trials are needed in both groups – that is really important. One confounding dilemma though, particularly in the USA, is that when people are getting to the end stages of a disease, there is difficulty in accepting this. I noticed from your data on Alzheimer disease that pneumonia was far and away the commonest cause of death. However, many people get pneumonia when they are tube fed. So there is confounding between overaggressive nutritional supplementation and getting pneumonia from a normal end-stage process. I wonder whether you have tried to differentiate those processes in your study? At some point it is acceptable to let somebody die, but in the USA we sometimes have trouble with that.

Dr. Vellas: In the ELSA study, we only had people with mild dementia, but in our special care unit we admit many people with severe dementia and this is one of our worst problems. What should we do with severely demented people who don't want to eat? If there is a solution, we think it is prevention: maintaining the nutritional status as long as possible by nutritional intervention.

Dr. Morley: I agree. There was a recent article from an Italian group [1] where they showed that with good feeding and good care in a nursing home, weight loss does not occur in Alzheimer patients. In our experience this is associated with a good quality of life. The secret is to do it early and to prevent weight loss rather than to come late in the day. When it is late, it is usually too late.

Reference

1. Franzoni S, Frisoni GB, Boffelli S, Rozzini R, Trabucchi M. Good nutritional oral intake is associated with equal survival in demented and non-demented very old patients. *J Am Geriatr Soc* 1996; 44: 1366–70.

Mini NutritionalAssessment (MNA): Research and Practice in the Elderly:
B. Vellas; P.J. Garry; Y. Guigoz (eds),
Nestlé Nutrition Workshop Series Clinical & Performance Programme, Vol. 1, pp. 93–100,
Nestec Ltd.; Vevey/S. Karger AG, Basel, © 1999.

Mini Nutritional Assessment and Cancer

Gilbert B. Zulian, Gabriel Gold[a], François Herrmann[a] and Jean-Pierre Michel

Cesco and [a] Geriatric Hospital, Department of Geriatrics, Geneva University Hospital, Thônex, Switzerland

Malignant diseases are among the leading causes of premature death in Western countries, and this is also becoming a tragic reality in other parts of the world [1]. Cigarette smoking is the major risk factor for cancers of the respiratory tract and the third most important risk factor for developing any type of cancer. Diet is considered to be the second highest risk factor for cancer, mostly in countries with high animal fat intake but also in those where vitamin deficiencies are common. Age remains the most important risk factor, and as the proportion of elderly people is rapidly increasing, the incidence of cancer is unlikely to decrease.

Preventive measures aimed at reducing tobacco consumption markedly influence the incidence of smoking-related diseases. Supplementation of nutritional deficits and dietary interventions might decrease the incidence of some cancers and improve the prognosis of others. In the Chinese province of Linxian, recent data have shown how efficient nutritional supplementation can be, with a 20% reduction in the incidence of esophageal and gastric cancers [2]. Vegetarians are believed to be 40% less likely to die of cancer in Great Britain than people who include meat in their diet, but these data have failed to reach clear-cut statistical significance [3]. In addition, decreasing the amount of animal fats in the diet of women with advanced breast cancer has resulted in an improvement in prognosis and better survival [4].

Reasons for considering nutritional assessment as an important step in the interdisciplinary approach to the management of patients with cancer are therefore multiple. Proper assessment includes a nutritional history (taking into account weight loss and concomitant diseases), a detailed physical examination, anthropometric measurements such as triceps skinfold thickness and mid arm muscle circumference, laboratory tests such as albumin or prealbumin and transferrin, immune function studies, and clinical expertise.

The Mini Nutritional Assessment (MNA) has been developed to detect malnutrition in elderly patients. It has been successfully validated in Toulouse and New Mexico, and it takes approximately 10 min for its 18 items to be completed [5]. It includes anthropometric measurements, a global assessment, a dietary questionnaire, and a subjective assessment. The MNA distinguishes adequate nutritional status (MNA score >24), risk of malnutrition (MNA score 17–23), and frank malnutrition (MNA score <17).

Recent data have shown an increased risk of malnutrition in a Hispanic elderly population of New Mexico and in some retirement homes in Belgium. In addition, 18% of home care elderly people living in Paris were found to be malnourished [6]. In nursing homes, the proportion is as high as 30–60% [7]. Finally, 15% of elderly people were found to be malnourished on hospital admission in Switzerland, as were 11% of elderly people receiving dialysis in Toulouse [6]. Further data are presently being collected on conditions such as anorexia and Alzheimer disease, in the preoperative setting, and as part of multidimensional geriatric assessment or as a tool for nutritional intervention.

In cancer patients, MNA could help determine the most appropriate diagnostic procedures and the best therapeutic strategies by identifying individuals at risk of malnutrition, and might provide an adequate tool to measure the efficacy of nutritional interventions. Before this stage, MNA must first be shown to be practical and reliable in an unselected population of elderly patients with cancer. Over a period of 12 months, we have introduced the MNA in the routine assessment of all patients admitted to both units of a university geriatric hospital, located in an urban area of 400,000 people.

Patients and Methods

From 1 January to 31 December 1996, all patients admitted to the Geriatric Department of Geneva University Hospitals were considered eligible for the study. The original MNA questionnaire was slightly adapted to our local practice. The 18 items were strictly similar but were put in a different order: global evaluation, diet information, subjective evaluation, and anthropometric measurements. The MNA was performed by a physician as part of the routine geriatric admission assessment. The completed questionnaire was included in the medical file. The ward dietician reviewed the results of the MNA, initiated dietary intervention when appropriate, and entered the MNA score into a computerized database. Serum albumin concentrations were also obtained and entered into the database. ANOVA test using the method of Kruskall-Wallis was used to compare the data obtained in cancer patients with those in noncancer patients.

Results

In all, 2,890 patients were admitted during the study period (2,283 at the Geriatric Hospital and 607 at the Cesco). MNA scores were available for 442 patients (15.3% of all admissions) and were fully completed in 387 cases (13.4%). Among the 607 patients with cancer admitted in 1996, MNA scores were available for 71 patients (11.7%) and were fully completed in 58 cases (9.5%). For the purpose of the study, only data obtained from the fully completed MNA forms in either cancer or noncancer patients were analyzed. There were thus 329 MNA forms in noncancer patients and 58 MNA forms in cancer patients.

Mean age was 84.2 ± 6.6 years for the whole group, 84.0 ± 6.6 years in the noncancer group, and 85.6 ± 6.3 years in the cancer group. There were 277 female patients and 109 males. In the noncancer group, there were 248 females and 80 males; in the cancer group there were 29 females and 29 males. There was thus a significant predominance of females in the noncancer group.

Cancer types were prostate (n = 13), breast (n = 10), hematological (n = 10), gastrointestinal tract (n = 9), skin (n = 8), brain (n = 6), respiratory tract (n = 5), urinary tract (n = 5), uterus (n = 2), and others (n = 3).

Overall MNA scores (mean ± SD) were 20.21 ± 4.13 in noncancer patients and 19.07 ± 3.89 in cancer patients. The difference is marginally significant (p = 0.0521). Further details on patient characteristics and MNA results are given in Table 1 for every measurable item.

Table 1. Patients' characteristics and results

	Cancer patients	Noncancer patients	*p* value
Number (males/females)	58 (29/29)	329 (80/248)	
Age, years	85.57	83.95	NS
MNA score	19.07	20.21	0.0521
Body mass index	23.40	23.93	NS
Brachial circumference, cm	23.96	24.59	NS
Calf circumference, cm	31.17	31.05	NS
Recent weight loss, kg	6.23	3.90	NS
Present weight, kg	60.31	58.87	NS
Knee-heel distance, cm	47.86	46.41	NS
Independence			
Yes	43	244	NS
No	15	85	
>3 drugs			
Yes	33	201	NS
No	25	128	
Acute disease or stress			
Yes	29	122	NS
No	29	207	

Table 1 (continued)

	Cancer patients	Noncancer patients	*p* value
Mobility			
Bedridden	6	38	NS
Home	18	84	
Normal	34	207	
Dementia			
Severe	3	22	NS
Moderate	23	132	
None	32	175	
Skin wounds			
Yes	10	41	NS
No	48	288	
Meals			
1	8	36	NS
2	15	75	
3	35	218	
Dairy products			
Yes	41	246	NS
No	14	74	
Eggs or vegetables			
Yes	43	258	NS
No	11	61	
Meat, fish, poultry			
Yes	42	253	NS
No	13	67	
Fruits or vegetables			
Yes	43	236	NS
No	15	93	
Anorexia			
Severe	4	13	NS
Moderate	17	72	
None	37	244	
Drinks			
<3	7	34	NS
3–5	28	173	
>5	23	122	
Eating			
With assistance	1	16	NS
Some difficulty	5	36	
No problem	52	277	
Malnourished			
Yes	0	6	NS
Moderately	17	66	
No	41	257	
Health			
Worse	22	82	NS
Good	8	59	
Not known	24	156	
Better	4	32	
Serum albumin, g/l	31.32	33.40	0.0163
Hospital duration, days	46.2	52.9	NS

Discussion

In this large group of unselected elderly patients referred to a University Department of Geriatrics, we found that MNA forms were inconsistently completed. Complete MNA scores were available for only 10% of all admissions. This raises several issues.

Time: The questionnaire was more time-consuming than expected. It has been reported that the MNA can be performed in 10 min. Although this may be the case when evaluating alert and cognitively intact elderly people, the experience reported by admitting physicians in our hospital was very different. Most patients were quite ill and one third presented with dementia or delirium. Collaboration was sometimes difficult to obtain. The MNA may require more time and effort in a frail, acutely ill, and cognitively impaired population.

Professionals involved: Nurses or dieticians could have greater motivation and more time to focus on nutritional status than the admitting physician. Most physicians receive little training in nutrition during medical school and may not understand the value of assessing nutritional status in acutely ill older individuals.

Location and timing: The admission ward may not have been the ideal location. A large amount of information must be obtained upon admission. Geriatric assessment is a long process and the nutritional evaluation may be omitted or deferred by a harried physician who does not always grasp its importance. However, only the admission ward includes single rooms in our hospital and provides a comfortable and quiet environment for assessing patients.

Cognitive impairment and lack of informants: Approximately one third of all patients on admission suffer from dementia and another third present with mild cognitive impairment. Unless family members or other informants are present, it may be particularly difficult to collect accurate and complete information on these cases.

We report a high percentage of malnourished patients. Although our results should be interpreted with great caution in view of the low MNA completion rate, they are consistent with other published reports of a 30–60% prevalence of nutritional impairment in elderly hospital inpatients [8–10].

We found a borderline statistically significant difference ($p = 0.0521$) in the total MNA scores between cancer patients and noncancer patients. However, it is unclear whether a total MNA score difference of one point is clinically meaningful. Our results are consistent with a similar nutritional status in both groups. Patient characteristics such as age, body mass index, brachial and calf circumference, weight, weight loss, and knee height were comparable in cancer and noncancer patients. In addition, none among the 18 items of the MNA questionnaire was found to reach a level of statistical significance. Our results do not take into account the type or stage of the cancer involved. It is likely that this information may be more closely associated with nutritional status than the simple presence or absence of a malignancy.

More importantly, a high proportion of patients in both groups was found to be at risk of malnutrition, with MNA scores between 17 and 23.5. These patients, whose nutritional risk often goes undetected, represent the largest group and may benefit the most from preventive interventions. Thus routine application of the MNA may be particularly useful in an elderly population referred to a general hospital.

We describe a significant association ($p = 0.0163$) between serum albumin concentrations and a diagnosis of cancer. This may reflect inflammation as well as nutritional status and should be interpreted accordingly. Since C-reactive protein was not measured routinely, we are unable to determine whether albumin concentrations reflect nutritional information not included in the MNA or whether the association described is related to inflammatory changes.

Conclusion

We have failed to show a striking difference between cancer patients and non-cancer patients using the MNA questionnaire as a diagnostic tool for malnutrition. This may in part be related to difficulties in obtaining complete MNA forms. Future research should be directed at developing a shorter questionnaire with perhaps no more than five to eight questions to screen elderly patients in the admission ward. Patients thus identified would then answer the full MNA questionnaire to confirm the initial findings. Nutritional interventions could then take place.

References

1. Magrath I, Litvak J. Cancer in developing countries: opportunity and challenge. *J Natl Cancer Inst* 1993; 85: 862–74.
2. Li JY, Taylor PR, Dawsey S, *et al.* Nutrition intervention trial in Linxian, China: multiple vitamin/mineral supplementation, cancer incidence, and disease-specific mortality among adults with esophageal dysplasia. *J Natl Cancer Inst* 1993; 85: 1492–8.
3. Thorogood M, Mann J, Appleby P, McPherson K. Risk of death from cancer and ischaemic heart disease in meat and non-meat eaters. *BMJ* 1994; 308: 1667–70.
4. Holm LE, Nordevang E, Hjalmar ML, *et al.* Treatment failure and dietary habits in women with breast cancer. J Natl Cancer Inst 1993; 85: 32–6.
5. Guigoz Y, Vellas BJ, Garry PJ. Mini nutritional assessment: a practical assessment tool for grading the nutritional state of elderly patients. *Facts Res Gerontol* 1994; 4 (suppl 2): 15–59.
6. Guigoz Y, Nourhashemi F, Vellas BJ. The MNA (mininutritional assessment): update. In: *Facts, research and intervention in geriatrics.* Paris: Serdi Publishing Co, 1997: 105–12.
7. Guigoz Y, Vellas B, Garry PJ. Assessing the nutritional status of the elderly: the mini nutritional assessment as part of the geriatric evaluation. *Nutr Rev* 1996; 54: S59–65.
8. Constans T, Bacq Y, Brechot JF, *et al.* Protein-energy malnutrition in elderly medical patients. *J Am Geriatr Soc* 1993; 40: 263–8.
9. Cederholm C, Hellerstrom K. Nutritional status in recently hospitalized and free-living elderly subjects. *Gerontology* 1992; 38: 105–10.
10. Rapin CH, Bruyere A, Romagnoli A, *et al.* L'alimentation des personnes âgées. *Méd Hyg* 1985; 43: 3517–22.

Discussion

Dr. Guesry: Dr. Zulian, you said that 58 MNA assessments were completed on 607 cancer patients (9.5%), whereas 229 were completed on 2,200 noncancer patients (10.4%), so there was a slight difference in the percentage completed. Don't you think there could be a bias in that when a very severe cancer patient arrives in hospital there may be a temptation to conclude that there are more urgent problems to solve than filling out an MNA form? That leads to the second question. Are you sure that the outpatient clinic or the emergency room is the best location to perform an MNA? I should have thought it would be better to wait a day or two and have a more relaxed atmosphere?

Dr. Zulian: I agree with you on your first point. The numbers are fairly small, the computer system was not working very well, and we might well have ended up with the wrong numbers. This is absolutely correct.

The second question depends on how you organize your hospital. In our hospital, the admission ward is the only place where the patients are in their own room, and when there is time to do the assessment. It would have been nice if the dieticians in our hospital had been interested in doing the assessment, but they weren't, nor were the nurses.

Dr. Arnaud-Battandier: Just to follow on what you said, do you have a program of renutrition for your cancer patients?

Dr. Zulian: No, we don't.

Dr. Griep: When you compared the MNA scores in cancer patients (19.07) and noncancer patients (20.21), there was borderline significance, with a p value of 0.054. Did you test these differences with the Mann-Whitney test, or did you just use the t test? I think that owing to the heterogeneity that we discussed before there might be some outliers in this dataset, and if you had used the Mann-Whitney test you might have found significance.

Dr. Zulian: The statistician who analyzed our results told me he only did the ANOVA test. I would be suspicious of trying to find a statistically significant difference in this dataset because I am not very confident of the data I presented to you.

*Dr. Griep:*But the Mann-Whitney test is particularly suited to this kind of data.

Dr. Zulian: I'll go back to the statistician and ask him if he wants to do that. Indeed, this was done later with the Wilcoxon-Mann-Whitney and a p value of 0.0324 was found but this is not adding any confidence to the data.

Dr. Schwenk: I'd like to commend Dr. Zulian for being so honest about the faults of his study. It is not common in conferences for people to admit to or even point out the faults of a study. My question is targeted more to the people who designed the MNA than to Dr. Zulian. The MNA was designed for healthy elderly people. Do you think that we should apply it unchanged to people with underlying chronic disease, or should we develop variances of the MNA targeted at this population? I would argue in favor of the second solution. As a clinician, I have to fill in a lot of forms, and I only tend to fill them in correctly if their result is of any use to me.

Dr. Vellas: The MNA was not designed for healthy elderly people, it was designed for frail elderly people. We know from various studies that geriatric assessment is very useful in frail elderly people. For very sick elderly people with severe malignancy the situation may be different. But for most frail elderly people the design of the MNA is appropriate.

Dr. Morley: Dr. Zulian's presentation on cancer is very important because among other things it shows that physicians do not care about nutrition. They will do all sorts of things, but they will not assess nutrition and they will not treat undernutrition. Again, this is one of the roles of MNA – as an educational tool, to make people more aware that nutrition does exist. The education process has to come with it, and we have to teach physicians how important it is. We must keep pushing forward and not worry too much about whether the MNA is absolutely perfect. It is a good teaching tool. If all it does is to teach people to be aware of nutrition I think we will be very lucky. I commend your study for showing just how hard it is, even in one of the major geriatric hospitals where people should be aware of nutrition, to get the message through. We all have the same problem.

Dr. Arnaud-Battandier: Do you have any plans for the future on nutrition?

Dr. Zulian: To show the data and try to identify people interested in promoting the message. Sometimes you have to consider politics. In Geneva, for instance, there is no nutrition program in the University Hospitals because we do not have an identified person interested in the subject – or an accepted person, which might be different. Not only do you need specialists, but you need specialists who are accepted by the others, and that's something we do not have at the present time.

Dr. Chumlea: A comment to Dr. Morley's point that physicians don't know a lot about nutrition. The other problem is that the number of fellowships in geriatric medicine in the United States is extremely small. So it's a combination of both.

Mini Nutritional Assessment (MNA): Research and Practice in the Elderly:
B. Vellas; P.J. Garry; Y. Guigoz (eds),
Nestlé Nutrition Workshop Series Clinical & Performance Programme, Vol. 1, pp. 101–116,
Nestec Ltd.; Vevey/S. Karger AG, Basel, © 1999.

Comprehensive Geriatric Assessment (CGA) and the MNA: An Overview of CGA, Nutritional Assessment, and Development of a Shortened Version of the MNA

Laurence Z. Rubenstein, Judith Harker, Yves Guigoz[a], and Bruno Vellas[b]

GRECC (Geriatric Research Education and Clinical Center), Sepulveda VA Medical Center, Los Angeles, Calif., USA; [a] Nestlé Research Center, Nestec Ltd., Lausanne, Switzerland; [b] Department of Internal Medicine and Clinical Gerontology, CHU Purpan-Casselardit, Toulouse, France

What Is Comprehensive Geriatric Assessment?

Comprehensive geriatric assessment (CGA) is a multidimensional interdisciplinary diagnostic process intended to determine a frail elderly person's functional capabilities and medical and psychosocial problems, in order to develop an overall plan for treatment and long-term follow-up. While CGA includes many components of the standard medical diagnostic evaluation, it focuses on the special needs of frail elderly persons. As such, CGA goes well beyond the routine examination in its emphasis on functional status and quality of life, its thoroughness, and its use of standardized measurement instruments and interdisciplinary teams [1].

CGA usually incorporates at least four broad assessment domains: medical status, functional status, psychological function, and socioenvironmental indices. Each domain contains a number of subdomains, and most are assessed with the assistance of standardized scales and instruments outlined in Table 1. For example, psychological function contains at least the major subdomains of cognition and affect, each of which can be assessed by a number of standardized scales (for example, the mini-mental state examination for cognition and the geriatric depression scale for affect). Medical status contains many subdomains corresponding to specific organ systems (for example, cardiac, pulmonary) as well as

Table 1. Measurable domains of comprehensive geriatric assessment with examples of possible measurement scales*

Domain/*subdomain*	Essential concepts	Examples of useful scales
Global functional status		
Basic activities of daily living (ADL)	Self-care, basic mobility, incontinence	Katz ADL, Lawton Personal Self-Maintenence Scale (PSMS), Barthel Index
Instrumental activities of daily living (IADL)	Household activities, shopping, finances, etc.	Lawton IADL, Older Americans Resources and Services (OARS) IADL section
Mental health		
Cognitive status	Cognition, mental function, memory, etc.	Folstein Mini-mental State (MMS), Kahn Mental Status Questionnnaire (MSQ)
Affective status	Depression, anxiety, well-being	Yesavage Geriatric Depression Scale (GDS), Zung Depression Scale
Social activities and supports	Social network, communitiy activities, etc.	Lubben Social Network Scale, OARS Social Resources Section
Physical function		
Mobility – gait and balance	Gait, balance, fall risk	Tinetti Perfomance-Oriented Mobility Assessment (POMA), Get-up & Go Test
Nutritional adequacy	Nutritional status and risk	Mini Nutrition Assessment (MNA), Nutrition Screening Initiative Checklist

* Adapted from Table 15-1 in Rubenstein LZ and Rubenstein LV [2].

functional groupings (for example, special senses, gait and balance). An important subdomain of medical status is nutritional status, and this too contains subcomponents. These are dealt with in detail elsewhere in this volume.

CGA is performed in a variety of locations and health care contexts, usually in conjunction with patient admission or enrollment in a program and often repeated or updated at periodic intervals thereafter. Not only is it a fundamental part of care on special geriatric inpatient units, but it is a basic part of most other specialized geriatric care programs (for example, home care, day hospital, rehabilitation programs, geriatric consultation services, community preventive health programs for seniors), occurring in conjunction with patient entry and often repeated or updated at periodic intervals thereafter. It is also performed in many primary care settings that care for older patients, as a supplement to the standard medical evaluation.

However, the process of CGA is not the same in all these settings and can vary considerably in complexity. It can be viewed as a continuum, ranging from a limited screening assessment by primary care physicians or community health workers focused on identifying an older person's functional problems and disabilities, to more thorough evaluation of these problems by a geriatrician or interdisciplinary team coupled with initiation of a therapeutic plan in specialized centers. Because it has become so much an integral part of care in these geriatric programs, it is often difficult to distinguish the benefits of the CGA process itself from those of the treatment, rehabilitation, and follow-up processes which follow the CGA and are often provided in the same settings. Indeed, when discussing CGA and its benefits, one usually considers CGA together with its entire geriatric care and follow-up program. This broader context of CGA creates both a challenge for interpretation and an opportunity for greater program success.

The Benefits of CGA

A growing body of literature supports the effectiveness of CGA programs in several different settings. Early descriptive studies of CGA programs in hospitals and the community indicated several important benefits, such as improved diagnostic accuracy, reduced discharges to nursing homes, increased functional status, and reduced drug treatment. However, these early studies did not have concurrent controls, and thus could not distinguish the effects of the programs from the simple effects of improvement over time. Nor was it clear how these apparent benefits, most of which affected process of care, would relate to longer-term outcome benefits.

Beginning in the 1980s, controlled studies began to emerge which corroborated some of the earlier descriptive studies and documented additional benefits to both process of care and to short- and long-term outcomes. Many of these controlled trials showed that programs led to improved survival, decreased use of institutional services, and improved levels of both mental and physical functioning. However, there was considerable diversity in trial results, with many showing a high degree of program benefit, while others reported minimal effects [2, 3].

To resolve some of this discrepancy, and to try to identify particular program elements associated with particular benefits, systematic meta-analysis has been performed [4]. This meta-analysis included published data from 28 controlled trials, as well as substantial amounts of previously unpublished data systematically retrieved from many of the studies. The meta-analysis subdivided CGA programs into five types: hospital units (n = 6 trials), hospital consultation teams (n = 8), in-home assessment services (n = 7), outpatient assessment services (n = 4), and "hospital-home assessment services" (n = 3), which performed in-home assessments on patients recently discharged from hospitals. The meta-analysis confirmed many of the major reported benefits for many of the program types. Among these statistically and clinically significant benefits included: reduced risk of mortality (by 22% for hospital-based programs at 12 months, and by 14% for all programs combined at 12 months); improved likelihood of living at home (by 47% for hospital-based programs and by 26% for all programs combined at 12 months); reduced hospital admissions (by 12% for all programs at study end); greater chance of cognitive improvement (by 47% for all programs at study end); and greater chance of physical function improvement for patients on hospital units (by 72% for hospital units). In general, hospital units and in-home assessment programs showed the strongest and greatest variety of benefits. Covariate analysis showed that programs with actual clinical control of medical recommendations (as opposed to simply making consultations) and those providing extended follow-up were more likely to be effective.

Studies published since the meta-analysis have been, in general, consistent with the earlier results. Ongoing studies are continuing to examine the benefits of CGA in different program models, attempting to define the essential elements, the most appropriate patients, and the most cost-effective combinations.

Who Benefits Most from CGA? The Need for Patient Targeting

Since CGA programs can be expensive interventions, and since clearly not all elderly persons can measurably benefit from CGA, it is important to identify criteria that will help identify persons most likely to be helped. These are often called "targeting criteria," since they are intended to use clinical information to direct or "target" the most appropriate patients to a given program. Ideally, targeting criteria should separate all potential patients into at least three groups: persons appropriate for the program, those too healthy or independent, and those too dysfunctional or with too poor a prognosis. Actually, this concept of targeting is really a triage function, no different for geriatrics than selecting patients for most other clinical interventions. Most surgical procedures, for example, have a specific list of indications and contraindications, which could be used to identify persons as "too sick," "too well," and "appropriate." However, the targeting process has gained more attention within geriatrics, perhaps because of the relative scarcity of geriatric resources and because geriatric services had formerly been less selective of patients.

The nature of the targeting criteria differs between programs, and should reflect program purposes, structure, and costs. For example, hospital-based CGA units aimed at specific groups of patients (for example, stroke patients, patients with hip fracture, patients expecting a long stay) need more stringent and specific criteria than do community outreach programs that provide CGA to independent and relatively healthy elderly persons. As a rule, relatively inexpensive screening-type programs require only general and inclusive criteria, intended to admit a large proportion of elderly persons, while expensive hospital rehabilitation programs need very selective criteria.

While most targeting criteria have been derived empirically from clinical judgment, trying to select patients who would be most likely to benefit from the program, clinical trials have in some cases been able to validate the usefulness of the criteria. For example, in the Sepulveda VA randomized trial of an inpatient CGA unit [5, 6], a two phased patient identification process used selection criteria based on clinical experience. Hospital patients who remained in the hospital 7 days after admission were first screened for inclusion criteria by non-physician research assistants, looking for "persistent medical, functional, or psychosocial problems interfering with discharge home." Patients so identified would next be screened for exclusionary criteria (for example, terminal illness, unstable medical condition) by the research assistant in consultation with a geriatric physician, who would then make the final decision. The criteria divided the screened population into several subgroups (for example, "appropriate" (about 10% of those screened), "too independent," "terminal," and so on), and group assignment was shown to predict major clinical outcomes (that is, death, discharge location, 1-year living location, nursing home use). Validation of these criteria was performed in several stages over subsequent years (see below).

In a Canadian trial of a hospital-based CGA consultation team, Hogan & Fox [7] subdivided all elderly hospital patients into seven categories, within 48 h of admission, based on function, mental status, and prognosis. This process identified 38% of patients for the CGA intervention (categories 3–5), while 49% were excluded as being too functional (categories 1 and 2), and 14% were excluded as being either totally dependent or terminal (categories 6 and 7). The clinical categories were shown to predict subsequent mortality, nursing home placement, and functional status measured on the Barthel scale. The CGA intervention was then tested by random assignment, and the intervention was shown to improve survival, function, and possibly utilization of services for the targeted subgroup of patients.

Some of the most precise criteria have come from retrospective subgroup analyses of controlled trials, since controlled trials can pinpoint subgroups of their study populations who were more (and less) likely to benefit from the intervention. In the Sepulveda geriatric evaluation unit (GEU) trial [8], the randomized study population was subdivided by potential baseline risk factors and examined for 1-year survival. Although virtually all subgroups showed some significant benefit or positive trends, some subgroups clearly benefited more than others. For example, patients with lower baseline scores in function and mental status showed a greater survival benefit than patients with higher baseline scores. Similarly, increased benefit was seen among patients with heart and lung diseases and those with better affect scores. To refine targeting criteria, subgroups of patients were sought who would survive only if assigned to the GEU. Two such groups were cardiac patients with primary "geriatric" and "rehabilitation" problems, and noncardiac patients with primary "medical" problems.

In a trial of a hospital geriatric assessment unit by Applegate *et al.* [9], randomized patients were further stratified by their perceived risk of nursing home placement (high *vs.* low risk). There were greater effects from the unit on low risk stratum patients in terms of survival and functional improvement and on high risk stratum patients in terms of nursing home placement. The authors concluded that the beneficial effects of hospital CGA units on mortality and function may be greatest for elderly hospital patients with "moderate illness and moderate functional impairment."

While benefit size and the specific subgroup criteria for patients expected to derive maximum benefit differ in the above studies, all of them clearly conclude that patients who benefit most tend to be those with some definable geriatric problem interfering with function, yet who do not have a prognosis so poor as to be essentially too late for improvement. Thus again we see the trichotomous subdivision of elderly patients.

The meta-analysis discussed earlier confirmed the importance of targeting criteria in producing beneficial outcomes in controlled trials of CGA [4]. In particular, when the use of explicit targeting criteria in a CGA trial was included as a covariate, targeting was correlated with an increase in CGA benefits among certain CGA subgroups. For example, among the hospital-based CGA studies, positive effects on physical function and likelihood of living at home at 12 months were greater in studies that excluded patients who were relatively "too healthy." A similar effect on physical function was seen in the institutional studies that excluded persons with relatively poor prognoses. The reason for this effect of targeting on outcome size lies in the ability of careful targeting to concentrate the intervention on patients who can benefit, without diluting the effect size with persons too ill or too well to show a measurable improvement. Future research is certainly needed to refine these targeting criteria and to better tailor specific criteria to specific programs.

Assessing Nutrition in CGA: The Role of the MNA and Development of A Short Form Version, the MNA-SF

Nutritional deficiency is a common and extremely serious problem in the elderly population. While the reported prevalence of nutritional deficiency depends greatly on definitions used and populations studied, its surprisingly high rates can be considered to have reached epidemic proportions. For example, using the definition of "decreased nutrient reserves," up to 15% of ambulatory outpatients, 35–65% of elderly hospital patients, and 25–60% of institutionalized older adults have been found to be malnourished [10, 11]. These prevalence data are described in more detail elsewhere in this volume.

It seems obvious that detection of both overt malnutrition and risk for undernutrition must be a vital objective of CGA. The need for both screening instruments and more definitive diagnostic tools is clear, and is reflected in the proliferation of nutrition screening and assessment recommendations and tools that have emerged in the past two decades. These have been described in detail elsewhere [10, 12]. Among the most recent and extensively tested is the Mini Nutritional Assessment (MNA). The MNA fulfills many of the definitional criteria of both screening and diagnostic measures. It was developed and validated on large representative samples of elderly persons, and has been shown to be clinically useful in a variety of populations and countries for better identifying persons at nutritional risk and for providing information on dietary habits useful in intervention planning [11]. On the other hand, it is somewhat long and complex in comparison with many other screening tools, and this may impede its widespread acceptance as a short screening tool, particularly in situations where the CGA must be both brief and inclusive of multiple domains. The entire MNA was designed to take less than 20 min to administer, and was recently described as taking "about 10 min" [13], which is certainly reasonable for a diagnostic test, especially in a research or academic center. However, even 10 min might be too long to expect a primary care physician to add onto an already busy schedule for the average elderly person, in view of the many other components that typically need to be included in the comprehensive assessment – most of which have been designed to be administered in under 5 min. Moreover, several questions on the MNA require special training (for example, the anthropometry) and others are relatively subjective, requiring judgments either from the patient or caregiver, both of which might impair diagnostic accuracy. Thus a short form version of the MNA, if it could retain much of the validity and usefulness of the longer form, seems to be a worthwhile goal.

We have attempted to produce such a short form version (the MNA-SF) using a stepwise simplification process of the full MNA, trying to retain questions of the highest estimated importance, ease of data collection, face validity, and correlation both with the total MNA score and with clinical judgment of nutritional status. Our intent was to preserve as much predictive accuracy as possible while decreasing the time and training needed to administer the screen. We based our effort on the original population database of largely frail elderly persons in Toulouse, France, on which the MNA was developed and tested. Our intention is to try to subsequently validate the MNA-SF on other populations and modify it as necessary.

In attempting to select a subgroup of questions that would be retained in the MNA-SF, we used the following guidelines. We selected items that correlated well with the full MNA score and had good individual diagnostic characteristics (that is, high sensitivity, specificity, and overall diagnostic accuracy), based on independent clinical assessment of nutritional status. We chose items that, as a set, had high internal consistency. But we tried to avoid items that seemed to have redundant content, that required special training to administer, that were particularly time-consuming, that involved difficult subjective recall, or that may have had problems with missing or "don't know" answers. Ultimately, our aim was to identify a subscale that would approach the accuracy of the full MNA yet be brief enough for widespread use as a screening tool. One advantage of the MNA over many other nutritional assessment instruments is that it does not rely on laboratory testing, and this advantage would be retained by the MNA-SF. The ability of the MNA to help plan therapeutic interventions by defining eating habits would be lost in the MNA-SF, but if the full MNA were to supplement the MNA-SF for persons identified as being at risk, then this disadvantage could be overcome.

Methods

We used patient data from the original population in Toulouse,France, on whom the MNA was developed – the Toulouse 1991. The population has been fully described elsewhere [11], but briefly it consisted of both a hospital inpatient geriatric population (n = 105) stratified into three groups by serum albumin (<3.0 g/dl, n = 35; 3.0–3.5 g/dl, n = 35; >3.5 g/dl, n = 35), and a healthy elderly population living in the community, recruited from a community prevention program (n = 50). Characteristics of the overall group of subjects (n = 155) included the following: 66% were female; mean age was 79 years (70% ≥75 years); 56% had a mini-mental state score of <24/30; 43% had an ADL score of <4/6; 49% reported moderate to severe anorexia; 45% were taking more than three drugs, and 56% had serum albumin of ≤3.5 g/dl. Thus the population was largely an ill and frail hospital population combined with a smaller group of healthy elders.

Data from the full MNA on the entire population had been entered into the database, with complete MNA data available for most (n = 151) of the population. As described elsewhere [11], the MNA consists of 18 questions in four categories: anthropometric measurements (four questions), global assessment (six questions), dietary assessment (six questions), and self-perception of health and nutrition (two questions). Individual questions have weighted scores, and the scale is scored from 0 to 30. Interpretation established for the total score is: ≥24 = well-nourished, 17–23.5 = at risk of malnutrition, <17 = undernutrition.

We began the simplification process by looking for possible redundancy of items. Pearson correlation coefficients were calculated between all pairs of items. Any items with very high inter-item correlation ($r > 0.80$) plus overlapping item content were considered redundant. Although some pairs of items had moderately high correlations, none was redundant.

Next we looked at internal consistency, using item analysis procedures (Systat 7.0 and Crunch 4.1), with the Cronbach's coefficient α as a measure of internal consistency. Although we recognized that nutritional status has multiple components, we assumed that these components measured aspects of a single underlying construct, namely nutritional status. Therefore the 18 items were treated as a single scale. These procedures report the α for all 18 items and, for each item, the change in α (for the remaining 17 items) if that item were excluded. If excluding an item produced no change or an increase in α, thereby increasing the overall internal consistency, that item was a candidate for exclusion from the item set. Successive calculations of internal consistency were done with the best remaining 15, 12, nine, and six items. As an independent check, Pearson correlations between each item and the MNA total score were examined. Items that had poor correlations to the total score were also candidates for exclusion, and the items selected were in agreement with those identified by item analysis. Finally we calculated the optimal sensitivity, specificity, and diagnostic accuracy for each item, using physician judgment of nutritional status (clinical status) as the gold standard. Items with poorest relation to clinical status were also candidates for exclusion. Again, there was good agreement with the candidates selected by item analysis.

After identifying what seemed to be the best possible short form version (MNA-SF), we tested the MNA-SF against the full MNA to see how much accuracy had been lost and to discover if there were items we might need to add back in order to improve the short form to an acceptable level. Sensitivity, specificity, and overall diagnostic accuracy for the MNA-SF were compared to those for the full MNA in ability to identify persons judged independently to have nutritional problems, as well as to identify persons with deficient serum albumin concentrations. Threshold values for the MNA-SF were chosen based on receiver-operating curves (ROCs) of diagnostic accuracy.

Results

Table 2 shows the diagnostic characteristics (sensitivity, specificity, overall predictive accuracy) of the 18 individual items of the MNA, using clinical nutritional status as the gold standard. The clinical status rating of "uncertain" (n = 13) was excluded from these calculations. χ^2 Analysis examined the relation of each item's response categories with clinical status (normal or malnourished). All but item No 5 were significant at $p < 0.05$. For items with the same number of response categories, the larger the χ^2, the stronger the relation. For all items with more than two response categories, classification cutpoints were selected to maximize sensitivity. In some cases, two cutpoints were tried – for example, with item No 1, we tested body mass index (BMI) values of both <21 and <23 as possible indicators of malnutrition.

As can be seen, individual items were quite variable in their ability to predict overall nutritional status, with some items being quite good, that is, No 1 (BMI), No 4 (weight loss), No 7 (illness/stress), No 8 (housebound), No 9 (dementia/depression), No 14 (appetite loss), and others not very good, for example, No 2

Table 2. Diagnostic characteristics of the individual 18 items from the MNA, relative to their ability to identify individuals with nutritional problems as determined by clinical diagnosis (as the gold standard), using the Toulouse 91 population database (n = 151)

Item	Content	Sensitivity	Specificity	Accuracy	χ^2 value
1*	BMI <23	0.795	0.774	0.787	53.058
2	Mid-arm circumference ⩽22	0.125	1.00	0.454	7.186
3	Calf circumference <31	0.614	0.960	0.745	45.821
4*	Recent weight loss >1 kg	0.875	0.774	0.837	62.690
5	Lives in NH or hospital	0.483	0.604	0.528	1.014 (n.s.)
6	Takes >3 Rx medications	0.584	0.755	0.648	15.379
7*	Acute illness/stress	0.910	0.906	0.909	92.556
8*	Housebound	0.775	0.925	0.831	67.787
9*	Dementia or depression	0.652	0.943	0.761	48.028
10	Pressure sores	0.416	0.981	0.627	26.694
11	<3 meals/day	0.122	0.962	0.489	7.346
12	<3 protein markers	0.588	0.736	0.645	15.174
13	<2 vegetables/day	0.165	1.00	0.486	9.715
14*	Appetite loss or eating problem	0.775	0.981	0.852	76.054
15	<5 cups fluid/day	0.565	0.792	0.652	17.479
16	Self-feeding difficulty	0.472	0.981	0.690	32.462
17	Self-rated malnutrition	0.652	0.962	0.768	51.331
18	Lower self-rated health status	0.618	0.887	0.718	35.915

* Indicates items selected for the MNA-SF.

(mid-arm circumference), No 5 (institutionalized), No 6 (takes >3 drugs), No 11 (has <3 meals/day), No 13 (has <2 fruits or vegetables/day). The six items with the highest sensitivity and overall accuracy were selected for the MNA-SF. A seventh item with good apparent accuracy, No 17 (self-rated malnourishment), was excluded because of a relatively large proportion (32/155: 21%) of "don't know" answers. Item No 3 (calf circumference) was not quite as sensitive or accurate as item No 9 and also had the problem of requiring some additional examination time and calculation. Item No 18 (self-rated health) was the next best item, but again was not as good as item No 9 and seemed to have less face validity. These procedures fortunately converged on the same set of six items as possible candidates for inclusion in the MNA-SF.

Figure 1 shows the correlation between the MNA-SF and the full MNA. As can be seen, the correlation is remarkably high (r = 0.969). Using a cutpoint for the MNA-SF of ≤10/14 as an indicator of possible malnutrition, all of the persons identified on the MNA as "malnourished" (MNA score <17) would have been picked up, as would all but two of those identified as "at risk" (MNA score 17–23). Thus, using the full MNA as the gold standard and setting the threshold at ≤10/14, the sensitivity of the MNA-SF for identifying "malnourished" or "at

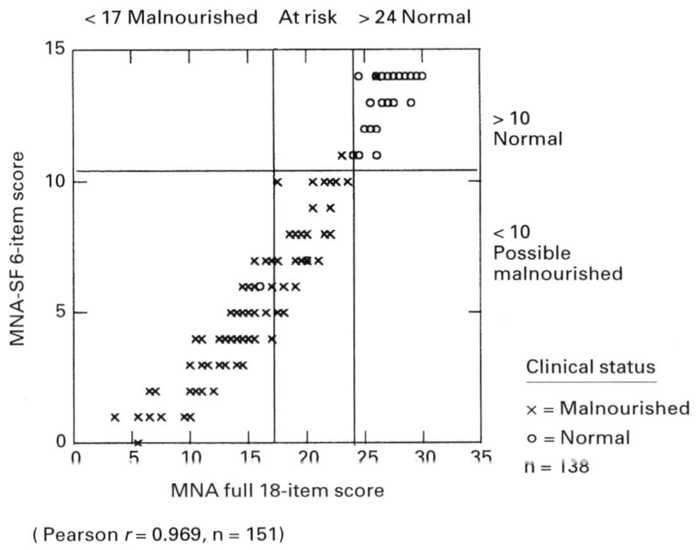

Fig. 1. Correlation between the six-item MNA-SF and the full 18-item MNA.

risk" persons is 97.9% (96/98), the specificity is 100% (53/53), and the overall predictive accuracy is 98.7%. (In fact, lowering the MNA-SF threshold to ≤7/14 would have still identified all the "malnourished" persons, but would have missed a substantial number of persons at risk.)

The correlation between the MNA-SF and serum albumin level is quite high ($r = 0.679$) – almost as high as that between albumin and the full MNA ($r = 0.699$). Moreover, the ability of the MNA-SF to identify subnormal albumin (<3.5 g/dl) is remarkably good. All but two persons with a subnormal albumin concentration were identified among the persons with MNA-SF scores of ≤10/14. Again, this gives an overall predictive accuracy of 98.7% in this population.

Table 3 shows the relative predictive accuracy of the full MNA and the MNA-SF with regard to recognizing persons with clinically determined definite or possible malnutrition, as well as persons with a serum albumin of <3.5 g/dl. With regard to predicting persons with clinical malnutrition, the full MNA has an overall predictive accuracy of 97.1%, versus a virtually indistinguishable 96.4% for the MNA-SF.

Table 3. Predictive accuracy of the full MNA and the MNA-SF for recognizing persons with clinical malnutrition (judged by an expert clinician) and persons with serum albumin of <3.5 g/dl

	Sensitivity	Specificity	Overall accuracy
Full MNA correctly identifying persons with clinical malnutrition threshold score <24/28	0.989	0.943	0.971
MNA-SF correctly identifying persons with clinical malnutrition threshold score <10/14	0.978	0.943	0.964
Full MNA correctly identifying persons with albumin <3.5 g/dl threshold score <24/28	0.976	0.761	0.881
MNA-SF correctly identifying persons with albumin <3.5 g/dl threshold score <10/14	0.954	0.764	0.871
Expert judgment as "malnourished or uncertain" ability to predict albumin <3.5 g/dl	0.988	0.764	0.890

As with any screening test, choice of threshold is crucial in determining the diagnostic characteristics. There is usually an inverse relation between sensitivity and specificity, and as the threshold for "normality" is lowered (that is, to include more persons as "abnormal") the sensitivity of the test increases, while the specificity decreases. This can be seen visually in Figure 2, and it can be seen that for the MNA-SF, the optimal threshold appears to be >10/14 as indicating "normal" or low risk.

Based on the above data, it seems very likely that the MNA-SF will be a good first step of a two-step screening strategy for nutritional problems, which would be followed by administration of the full MNA to persons identified as potentially at risk by the MNA-SF. Assuming the population screened was similar to the largely frail one employed here, this two-step strategy would result in a 34% reduction in persons needing to receive the full MNA, since 34% of the Toulouse 1991 population had a MNA-SF score of >10/14. If, as is likely, the population to be screened in many geriatric settings was more independent, then a much higher proportion of people would be screened out by the MNA-SF, and the savings would be substantially greater.

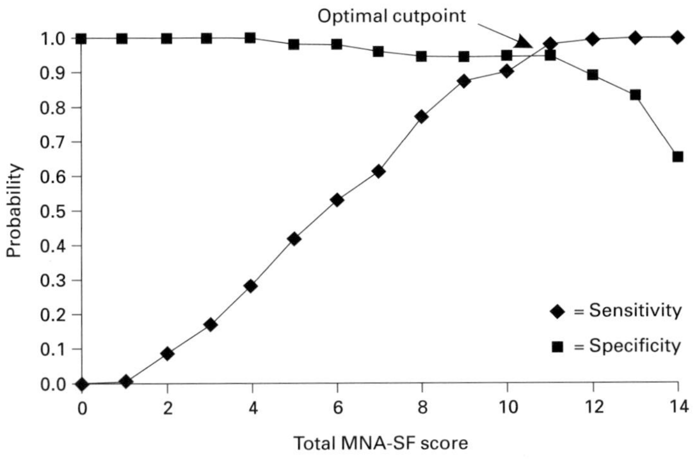

Fig. 2. Choosing a threshold (cutpoint) on the MNA-SF for identifying persons with nutritional problems.

Discussion

Assuming that screening for nutritional problems is a worthwhile strategy, it is apparent that the MNA can successfully uncover these problems, being highly correlated with both clinical assessment of nutritional status and with objective indicators such as serum albumin. However, in view of the large amount of information that needs to be collected in the course of the CGA, or even the geriatric screening process, a shorter form than the full MNA, if still accurate, would have real advantages. In this data analysis, we have been able to reduce the size and complexity of the MNA into a shortened form (MNA-SF), which retains most of the beneficial qualities of the original version, at least when the original population is examined.The resultant MNA-SF has six questions (as compared with the original 18) with a score range of 0 to 14, and eliminates most of the most time-consuming items (for example, anthropometric measurements) and questions asking for subjective judgments. It can be administered in approximately 3 min, as opposed to the estimated 10 min for the full MNA. It has a high correlation with both the full MNA ($r = 0.969$) and with serum albumin ($r = 0.679$ *vs.* 0.699 for the full MNA), and has high concordance with global assessment of nutritional status as being "malnourished *vs.* normal" (96.4% concordance *vs.* 97.1% for the full MNA). Moreover, using a cutpoint of 10/14, the MNA-SF has a sensitivity of 97.9%, a specificity of 100%, and an overall predictive accuracy of 98.7% for predicting malnutrition, using the full MNA as the gold standard.

Some caution is needed before extrapolating these data. First, the MNA-SF was developed and tested on the same population in which the original MNA was developed and tested. The MNA-SF needs to be validated on other populations. While it is likely that its screening characteristics will be even better among lower risk subjects, this speculation must be verified.

A major underlying assumption is that patients found to be malnourished or at risk will be able to benefit from being detected. In reality, it is unclear what proportion of malnourished persons discovered would really be able to benefit by being worked up and/or given nutritional counselling and supplementation, and what proportion are malnourished because of an underlying nonreversible medical condition. To answer this question, we are in desperate need of intervention studies. However, most clinicians in this area are not waiting for the study results, so convincing is the argument for attempting intervention in persons at clear nutritional risk. While treatment will only correct a subgroup of persons discovered to have malnutrition, unless these persons are discovered – probably through a screening or assessment process – this subgroup, regardless of size, is unlikely to benefit.

We must identify a rational strategy for providing nutritional screening in the population. The MNA can certainly be an important part of this strategy. Based on data presented here, it appears that the nutritional screening and assessment can be made even more efficient, and kept just as effective, by using this MNA-SF as the first step in a two-step screening process, which would then be followed up by using the full MNA or other techniques to help confirm the diagnosis and help plan specific treatment for appropriate persons. This strategy must next be tested by first validating the diagnostic characteristics of the MNA-SF itself on different populations, and then, if validated, studying this two-step strategy in clinical trials.

References

1. Rubenstein LZ, Wieland D, Bernabei R, eds. *Geriatric assessment technology: the state of the art.* Milan: Kurtis Publishers, 1995.
2. Rubenstein LZ, Rubenstein LV. Multidimensional geriatric assessment. In: *Brocklehurst's textbook of geriatric medicine.* London: Churchill Livingstone, 1997, ch 15.
3. Rubenstein LZ, Goodwin M, Hadley E, Rempusheski VF, Reuben DB, Winograd CH. Working group recommendations: targeting criteria for geriatric evaluation and management research. *J Am Geriatr Soc* 1991; 39: 37–41S.
4. Stuck AE, Siu AL, Wieland GD, Adams J, Rubenstein LZ. Comprehensive geriatric assessment: a meta-analysis of controlled trials. *Lancet* 1993; 342: 1032–6.
5. Rubenstein LZ, Josephson KR, Wieland GD, English P, Sayre JA, Kane RL. Effectiveness of a geriatric evaluation unit: a randomized clinical trial. *N Engl J Med* 1984; 311: 1664–70.

6. Rubenstein LZ, Josephson KR, Wieland GD, Kane RL. Differential prognosis and utilization patterns among clinical subgroups of hospitalized geriatric patients. *Health Serv Res* 1986; 20: 881–95.
7. Hogan DB, Fox RA. A prospective controlled trial of a geriatric consultation team in an acute-care hospital. *Age Ageing* 1990; 19: 107–13.
8. Rubenstein LZ, Wieland GD, Josephson KR, Rosbrook B, Sayre J, Kane RL. Improved survival for frail elderly inpatients on a geriatric evaluation unit: who benefits? *J Clin Epidemiol* 1988; 41: 441–9.
9. Applegate WB, Miller ST, Graney MJ, *et al.* A randomized controlled trial of a geriatric assessment unit in a community rehabilitation hospital. *N Engl J Med* 1990; 322: 1572–8.
10. Reuben DB, Greendale GA, Harrison GG. Nutrition screening in older persons. *J Am Geriatr Soc* 1995; 43: 415–25.
11. Vellas BJ, Guigoz Y, Garry PJ, Albarede JL, eds. *The Mini Nutritional Assessment: MNA,* 3rd ed. Paris: Serdi Publishing Co, 1997.
12. Vellas BJ, Guigoz Y. Nutritional assessment as part of the geriatric evaluation. In: Rubenstein LZ, Wieland D, Bernabei R, eds. *Geriatric assessment technology: the state of the art.* Milan: Kurtis Publishers, 1995: 179–94.
13. Faisant C, Lauque S, Guigoz Y, *et al.* Nutrition assessment and MNA. *Nutrition Intervention and the Elderly.* Paris: Serdi Publishing Co, 1997: 157–61.

Discussion

Dr. Morley: We have also seen that the MNA is very useful in preoperative evaluation, identifying those people who are malnourished but otherwise look healthy. We have seen that the MNA may play a prospective role in telling us what will happen in the nursing home. We have seen in intervention studies that the MNA may be useful to follow people, and we see that it taps into the cost of care in hospitals. So we have covered a large number of areas. Dr. Rubenstein, I'll ask you the first question. When you look at the short form of the MNA, how does it compare with the nutritional screening index that has been developed by another nutritional company in the USA? It seems very similar and could almost be used as a pre-screen. Have you had an opportunity to compare your short form of the MNA with the nutritional screening index?

Dr. Rubenstein: No, I haven't compared those two.

Dr. Morley: But how do you feel about the nutritional screening index as a tool that people can use in the community, before they get to a dietician or anyone else? It has a high sensitivity, but very poor specificity. It looks as though your short form may have better specificity and could be given to people to self-report.

Dr. Rubenstein: I really need to compare the two side by side. I think that the other screening test, which was not based on a more comprehensive assessment, may have omitted two or three items that are important. But I would like to check on that.

Dr. Schweizer: You mentioned that the upside of this is that you only need 2 min instead of 10 to carry it out. This may of course decrease or overcome the reluctance of people to use such assessments, as mentioned by Dr. Zulian. The downside, of course, is that you will lose a lot of information that could help you afterwards to design an intervention and to help those patients individually. You say that for two thirds of the patients who would maybe need such an intervention, you would add the full MNA. But my quick calculation shows that the resulting time gain is not very impressive. For 100 patients you would need 1,000 min for a full MNA, and with the combination of short form for all and a full MNA for two thirds, you would need nearly 900 min. Can you comment on that?

Dr. Rubenstein: Your point is well taken. For the frail population there is not so much saving if the two-step strategy is applied. The real savings come with its use as a screening test in a general elderly population. In that setting – and we'll see how it holds up in the New Mexico data and in some of the other databases – the benefits are the major time savings.

Dr. Vellas: An important point in geriatric assessment is that we don't have to use the same tool in healthy or frail elderly people. For a nutritional assessment, we need to use the MNA for frail elderly people, but for healthy elderly people, a short form test would be satisfactory.

Dr. Arnaud-Battandier: Following up on that, we find that in France general practitioners said they don't have time to do the MNA in all their elderly patients in their offices. So we are currently testing a list of 12 items which can be answered in 1 min: questions like do they have a disease, have they lost some weight, or do they live alone, etc., and if two of the risk factors are present, the doctor should do the full MNA.

Dr. Camilla: I found Dr. Rubenstein's intervention very useful. We really need an easy tool for primary care physicians to use in the primary care situation, and we need to be able to educate them into implementing a more comprehensive evaluation.

Mini Nutritional Assessment (MNA): Research and Practice in the Elderly:
B. Vellas; P.J. Garry; Y. Guigoz (eds),
Nestlé Nutrition Workshop Series Clinical & Performance Programme, Vol. 1, pp. 117–121,
Nestec Ltd.; Vevey/S. Karger AG, Basel, © 1999.

The Mini Nutritional Assessment for Preoperative Nutritional Evaluation: A Study on 419 Elderly Surgical Patients

Robert Cohendy

Département d'Anesthésie-Réanimation (Prof. J.-J. Eledjam), Centre Hospitalier Universitaire de Nîmes, France

Aging and malnutrition are both well-known surgical risk factors. With regard to age, several clinical studies have shown increased postoperative morbidity and mortality in patients over 60 or 65 years [1–4]. Malnutrition is also a well-identified risk factor [5–9]. However, studies specifically dealing with malnutrition in geriatric surgical patients are rather scarce [10–12] and none have used the Mini Nutritional Assessment (MNA). A descriptive study was therefore designed to assess the degree of malnutrition in elderly surgical patients using the MNA, which is known to be a practical tool for grading the nutritional state of elderly patients [13]. It was to be used for the routine evaluation of a surgical population of outpatients over 60 years of age seen on preoperative anesthesia consultation.

Methods and Patients

Patients

Every ambulatory patient over 60 seen on preoperative anesthesia consultation and scheduled for elective surgery was assessed. The following were not included: patients under 60 years of age; hospital inpatients (but institutionalized patients seen as outpatients were included); and patients admitted urgently or for emergency surgery. The evaluation was performed at two sites: a university affiliated public hospital (Centre Hospitalier Universitaire de Nîmes, France), and a private surgical hospital (Clinique Beau Soleil, Montpellier, France).

Table 1. American Society of Anesthesiologists (ASA) classification

ASA class	Disease state
1	No organic, physiologic, biochemical or psychiatric disturbance
2	Mild to moderate systemic disturbance that may or may not be related to the reason for surgery
3	Severe systemic disturbance that may or may not be related to the reason for surgery
4	Severe systemic disturbance that is life-threatening with or without surgery
5	Moribund patient who has little chance of survival but is submitted to surgery as a last resort (resuscitative effort)

Assessment of Nutritional Status

The MNA was applied by the anesthesiologist seeing the patients for preoperative evaluation. It was included in the overall clinical assessment, which routinely involved use of the American Society of Anesthesiologists (ASA) physical status score (Table 1). This score is widely used by anesthesiologists and the scores have been shown to be consistent between trained physicians [14]. The following were also recorded: gender, age, height, weight, body mass index (BMI), and type of scheduled operation, in four groups: orthopedics, digestive surgery, digestive endoscopy, and miscellaneous (mostly cataract operations). The MNA forms were filled in on site by the anesthesiologist seeing the patients. They were checked by a single investigator who was not involved in the clinical management of the patients. This investigator obtained or rectified the missing or ambiguous information, and calculated the MNA score.

Statistics

We used the following statistical tests as appropriate: Student's t test, χ^2 test, and nonparametric tests, with a critical probability (p) value set at 0.05. The results are given as median and range.

Results

Data on 419 patients seen between January and October 1996 were recorded. Their age, height, weight, and BMI values are given in Table 2. There were equal numbers of men and women, and the median age for the two genders was the same.

One hundred and ninety-one patients were seen in Montpellier and 228 in Nîmes (total = 419). Of those seen before elective surgery, 263 patients (62.8%) were scheduled for digestive surgery, 95 (22.7%) for orthopedic surgery, 28 (6.7%)

Table 2. Description of the 419 patients studied (median and range)

Age, years	Height, cm	Weight, kg	BMI, $kg \cdot m^{-2}$
72	165	68.5	25.2
60–98	134–186	34–114	12.8–40.4

BMI = Body mass index.

Table 3. MNA score: median and range (n = 408)

Anthropometric assessment	Global evaluation	Dietetic assessment	Subjective assessment	MNA score
7	8	8	3	29
0–8	0–9	0–9	0–4	1.5–30

Table 4. Distribution of ASA scores within the population studied: relation to the MNA score

	ASA1	ASA2	ASA3	ASA4	Overall
Number of patients	82	212	115	10	419
Percentage	19.6	50.6	27.4	2.4	100
MNA					
Median	27.5	26	24	19.5	26
Range	15–30	8.5–30	1.5–30	11–27	1.5–30

for digestive endoscopies, and 33 (7.9%) for miscellaneous reasons. In 82 cases the ASA score was 1 (19.6% of the total), in 212 cases it was 2 (50.6 %), in 115 cases it was 3 (27.4%), and in 10 cases it was 4 (2.4%). As expected, no patient was classified as ASA 5. In these patients, the median MNA score was 26, ranging from 1.5 to 30. In 11 cases the MNA score could not be calculated. Because the MNA score is the sum of four items, these were also recorded for each patient (Table 3). With regard to the nutritional thresholds, 28 patients (6.9% of the total) were found to have frank malnutrition (score less than 17), 104 (25.5%) were found to be at risk for malnutrition (MNA score between 17 and 23.5), and 276 (67.6%) were well nourished. The patients scheduled for digestive surgery had a significantly lower median MNA score (25.5, range 1.5–30), and there were fewer well-nourished patients (62%).

There was a strong relation between malnutrition and ASA score (Table 4). Moreover, among the 290 ASA 1–2 patients, 24.8% were found to be at least at risk of malnutrition, in contrast with 49.1% of at-risk and frankly undernourished patients in the group of 118 ASA 3–4 patients (χ^2 test, $p = 10^{-4}$).

Discussion

Among 419 ambulatory geriatric patients evaluated for elective surgery, the median MNA score was 26, ranging from 1.5 to 30, and about one third (32.4%) were at risk of malnutrition or frankly undernourished.

The population studied consisted of outpatients over 60 years of age seen in a teaching hospital as well as in a private surgical clinic. To avoid causing the nutritional results to be skewed, hospital inpatients and patients admitted urgently or for emergency surgery were not included. We therefore believe that the patients studied should have been representative of the geriatric surgical population as a whole, and that the clinical setting should have given a picture of current clinical practice. However, only half of the surgical patients were women, a smaller proportion than in a companion study performed in Nîmes during the same period on 1,337 elderly hospital inpatients, in which two thirds were women, and those subjects were also older (median age 84 years, range 55–103) [Compan B, personal communication].

Even in our relatively healthy population (two thirds of the patients were considered at low or mild risk for anesthesia and surgery), about one third of the patients were found to be at least at risk of malnutrition. Our population thus seemed to differ from those of other studies. For example, 10–15% of the surgical patients studied by Sandstrom *et al.* [16] and 3–12% of the patients in a meta-analysis on perioperative nutrition data by Detsky *et al.* [6] were not well nourished. As those studies were not specifically aimed at older patients, it seems that surgical patients over 60 years are most at risk of malnutrition.

In the particular setting of preoperative evaluation, the role of the ASA score should be considered. Though there appeared to be a close relation between the ASA and MNA scores, the ASA score alone obviously could not predict malnutrition. This shows that a clinical evaluation by a trained anesthesiologist takes into account at least some features relevant to the nutritional state of the patient, but also that such an evaluation is insufficient for a proper assessment of malnutrition and therefore inadequate for making a decision on preoperative nutritional intervention. It could be argued that the finding that the patients with the poorest preoperative prognosis are the most often undernourished is hardly surprising, but the fact that about half of the ASA 3 and 4 patients were at least at risk of malnutrition suggests that the ASA score could be used to screen surgical patients with regard to their nutritional status. This could have application for studies dealing with perioperative clinical nutrition of elderly patients in order to narrow their focus to those with the poorest prognosis, but we think it could also have a clinical application.

In conclusion, the MNA seemed useful for the preoperative evaluation of nutritional status. However, a comparison in this particular setting with other assessment tools, such as the subjective global assessment [17] or the nutritional risk index [5] remains to be done. Its effectiveness could be best judged by clinical studies relating the MNA score to the postoperative course of elderly patients, with or without the intervention of a perioperative nutritional program.

References

1. Barlow AP, Zarifa Z, Shillito RG, *et al.* Surgery in a geriatric population. *Ann R Coll Surg Engl* 1989; 71: 110–14.
2. Edwards AK, Seymour DG, McCarthy JM, Crumplin MKH. A 5-year survival study of general surgical patients aged 65 years and over. *Anaesthesia* 1996; 51: 3–10.
3. Gluck R, Munoz E, Wise L. Preoperative and postoperative evaluation of surgical patients. *Am J Surg* 1988; 155: 730–4.
4. Stephen CR. The risk of anesthesia and surgery in the geriatric patient. In: Krechel SW ed. *Anesthesia and the geriatric patient.* Orlando: Grune & Stratton, 1984: 231–46.
5. Buzby GP, Mullen JL, Matthews DC, Hobbs CL, Rosato EF. Prognosis nutritional index in gastrointestinal surgery. *Am J Surg* 1980; 139: 160–7.
6. Detsky AS, Baker JP, O'Rourke K, Goel V. Perioperative parenteral nutrition; a meta-analysis. *Ann Intern Med* 1987; 107: 195–203.
7. Di Costanzo J. Influence de l'état nutritionnel préoperatoire sur la morbidité postopératoire. *Nutr Clin Métab* 1995; 9: 39–44.
8. Mullen JL, Buzby GP, Matthews DD, Smale BF. Reduction of operative morbidity and mortality by combined preoperative and postoperative nutritional support. *Ann Surg* 1980; 192: 604–13.
9. The Veterans Affairs Total Parenteral Nutrition Cooperative Study Group. Perioperative total parenteral nutrition in surgical patients. *N Engl J Med* 1991; 325: 525–31.
10. Bastow MD, Rawlings J, Allison SP. Benefits of supplementary tube feeding after fractured neck of the femur: a randomised controlled trial. *BMJ* 1983; 287: 1589–92.
11. Delni M, Rapin CH, Bengoa JM, Delmas PD, Vasey H, Bonjour JP. Dietary supplementation in elderly patients with fractured neck of the femur. *Lancet* 1990; 335: 1013–16.
12. Seymour DG, Vaz FG. A prospective study of elderly general surgical patients. II. Post-operative complications. *Age Ageing* 1989; 18: 316–26.
13. Guigoz Y, Vellas B, Garry PJ. The Mini Nutritional Assessment (MNA): a practical assessment tool for grading the nutritional state of elderly patients. *Facts Res Gerontol* 1994; 4 (suppl 2): 15–59.
14. Owens WD, Felts JA, Spitnage EL. ASA physical status classification: a study of consistency of ratings. *Anesthesiology* 1978; 49: 239–43.
15. McWhirter JP, Pennington CR. Incidence and recognition of malnutrition in hospital. *BMJ* 1994; 308: 945–8.
16. Sandstrom R, Drott C, Hyltander A, *et al.* The effect of postoperative intravenous feeding (TPN) on outcome following major surgery evaluated in a randomized study. *Ann Surg* 1993; 217: 185–95.
17. Baker JP, Detsky AS, Wesson DE, *et al.* Nutritional assessment. A comparison of clinical judgment and objective measurements. *N Engl J Med* 1982; 306: 969–72.

Mini Nutritional Assessment (MNA): Research and Practice in the Elderly:
B. Vellas; P.J. Garry; Y. Guigoz (eds),
Nestlé Nutrition Workshop Series Clinical & Performance Programme, Vol. 1, pp. 123–130,
Nestec Ltd.; Vevey/S. Karger AG, Basel, © 1999.

The Mini Nutritional Assessment in Clinical Practice

Antoni Salvá, M. José Bleda[a] and Ignasi Bolibar[a]

Centre Geriàtric Cabanelles, PASS, Mataró, Barcelona, Spain; [a] Institut de Recerca Epidemiològica i Clínica, PASS, Mataró, Barcelona, Spain

The prevalence of protein-energy malnutrition (PEM) is very high among the elderly hospital inpatient population and among elderly people living in nursing homes. Some investigators estimate that between 30% and 60% of all such individuals are undernourished [1–3]. The outcome in these elderly people is worse if they have PEM and they also account for the largest number of hospital admissions and the highest morbidity and mortality [4–7]. The proportion of undernourished individuals in the community-based elderly population is lower. However, deficiencies in the intake of specific nutrients, and to a lesser extent of total energy intake, have been found through dietary surveys [8]. This is specially true in the case of frail elderly people.

For this reason, there is strong interest in developing methods of nutritional assessment that will allow rapid but precise screening and diagnosis [9], and which can easily be integrated into the various geriatric assessment programs. Normally, dietetic surveys, anthropometric evaluation, and biochemical assessments have been used for nutritional evaluation [10–12]. Recently, Guigoz *et al.* [13] developed a tool for nutritional assessment – the Mini Nutritional Assessment (MNA) – which includes 18 items in four different sections: anthropometry, global assessment, dietetic assessment, and subjective evaluation. This tool, validated for the geriatric population, allows people to be analyzed and classified according to their nutritional status into three groups: well-nourished, at risk of malnutrition, or malnourished. The test procedure allows the information to be collected in a systematic and objective way and makes follow-up easy, as well as facilitating comparison of results from other people or groups.

The elderly population is extremely heterogeneous. We find people with different levels of health, different levels of functional autonomy, and different social

Table 1. General characteristics of the patients under study

	1 Convalescence	2 Nursing home	3 Community
n	114	87	199
Sex, f:m	62:52	69:18	114:85
Age, years			
f	78.5 (8.4)	83.3 (8.2)	72.75 (5.5)
m	77.1 (10.8)	78.8 (9.5)	71.41 (5.1)
ADL			
0–1	52 (45.6)	9 (10.3)	0
2–4	41 (36.0)	23 (26.4)	0
5–6	21 (18.4)	55 (63.2)	199 (100)

f = Female; m = male.

and family situations. Some live in nursing homes. The use of validated tools such as the MNA can help us to understand and compare these different groups better from a nutritional perspective. In addition, at an individual level and in everyday clinical practice, correct and systematic nutritional evaluation will facilitate the development of preventive and therapeutic programs.

The aim of this chapter is to show some results relating to MNA assessment in three different samples of elderly subjects, living in convalescence geriatric units (CGUs), nursing homes, and in the community. The populations under study were from the city of Mataró (Barcelona, Spain).

The Spanish version of the MNA was obtained by translating the original French version and verifying the translation by the translation-retrotranslation method carried out by a bilingual person [14]. The MNA was administered by previously trained nurses. Any questions which the patient could not answer were answered by their main caregiver.

Other variables included in the study were: the activities of daily living (ADL), evaluated by the Katz scale [15]; cognitive impairment (only in the community-based study), measured by the Pfeiffer's test [16]; and finally, anthropometric variables, measured as basic indicators of nutritional status: weight, height, and body mass index (BMI), weight loss during the last three months, and serum albumin.

The three groups of elderly people under study were characterized as follows:

1 Convalescent Group
This group included people admitted to the CGU during 1995 (n = 114). There were 62 women and 52 men, mean age 78.5 (SD 8.4) and 77.1 (10.8) years, respectively. These were people in the subacute phase of a disease or in the rehabilitation process. As can be seen from Table 1, only 18.4% were indepen-

dent on the basis of the ADL assessment; in 24.4% the BMI was <21 and in 57.0% it was >23; 47% had a serum albumin of >35 g/l, 33% between 30 and 35 g/l, and 20% <30 g/l.

2 Nursing Home Group
This group included people who were admitted to the nursing home of Saint Joseph in Mataró in 1995 (n = 87). There were 69 women and 18 men, mean age 83.3 (8.2) and 78.8 (9.5) years, respectively. They did not have any acute disease at the time of the evaluation. Of these subjects, 63% were independent in five or six activities in the ADL assessment (Table 1); in 11.5% the BMI was <21 and in 73.6% it was >23; 84% had a serum albumin of >35 g/l, 15% between 30 and 35 g/l, and 1% <30 g/l.

3 Community Group
This group was a representative sample of people aged between 65 and 85 years, living in the city of Mataró (n = 199). There were 114 women and 85 men, mean age 72.75 (5.5) and 71.41 (5.1) years, respectively. All were independent as judged by the ADL assessment, and made less than three mistakes in the Pfeiffer test (Table 1; these were criteria for inclusion in the study). In only 1.5% was the BMI <21; in 95% it was >23.

The Mini Nutritional Assessment

As expected, the results of the MNA differed according to the group under study: 33.0% of subjects in the CGU, 5.7% in the nursing home, and only 0.5% in the community group fell into the *undernourished* category; 12.3% of the CGU group, 47.1% of the nursing home group, and 89.9% of the community group fell into the *well-nourished* category; and 54.4% of the CGU group, 47.1% of the nursing home group, and 9.5% of the community group fell into the *at-risk* category (Fig. 1).

The results obtained can be explained by the different health status of the groups at the time of evaluation. Patients admitted to convalescence units have had recent acute illnesses or are still in the process of recovery. Most have recent loss of independence which is responsible for their admittance. We have previously described the characteristics of people admitted to our CGU [17]. There is a significant variation in nutritional indices in these patients [4, 17], mainly because of the presence of inflammatory pathology, which results in anorexia (40% of our patients were reported to suffer from anorexia) and a decrease in nutritional intake. The low total score obtained from MNA in this group was mainly the result of the low scores in the anthropometric and dietetic assessments, which probably reflect their loss of appetite, reduced dietary intake, and resulting weight loss. The median value for the MNA in the original validation study [13] was 19.3 for people admitted to a geriatric unit, whereas it was 18.5 for the same population in our study. In other studies carried out in geriatric units, the re-

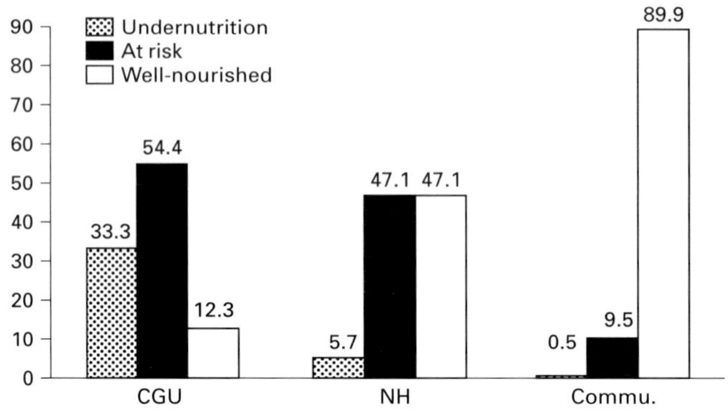

Fig. 1. Results of the MNA in the different groups. CGU = Convalescence geriatric unit; NH = nursing home; Commu = community.

ported malnutrition rates range from 10% to 15% – lower than in our population or in the original Toulouse study. The percentages of the population at risk always range between 33% and 62% [18, 19].

Those patients who are admitted in a nursing home without any acute diseases have characteristics which favor the appearance of nutritional problems [3]. Other studies are in agreement with respect to proportions of people classified by the MNA as being at risk of malnutrition – around 47–49% [14, 19]. The percentage of people classified as malnourished in the same studies ranged from 6% to 17%. In our group, this result reflected low scores for the global and subjective assessments. This proves the importance of risk factors in nursing homes.

Finally, we studied a population group in the community with a satisfactory health level. All these individuals were self-sufficient in performing ADL and they had good cognitive levels. Our results are similar to those from other studies carried out among outpatients, with the malnourished proportion ranging from 0% [18] to 3% in the Albuquerque study [13]. We only found one person with malnutrition criteria on MNA, but 18 (9.5%) were considered to be at risk (compared with 18% [13], 12% [19], and 3% [18] in other studies). The median MNA score in our population was 27. In the Albuquerque study, which was also community-based, the median was 25. The satisfactory levels of physical and cognitive function (which were criteria for inclusion in our study) show a population in good general health. The percentages of similar people classified as well-nourished in previous studies range from 80% in the Pertoldi study [18] to 97% in the Guigoz study [19].

Table 2. Correlation between total and partial MNA results and nutritional assessment variables

	Anthropometric area	Global assessment	Dietetic intake	Subjective assessment	Katz index	Albumin	BMI		Weight loss
							weight loss	no weight loss	
Total MNA NH	0.43	0.79	0.48	0.67	0.38	0.12	0.69	0.06	0.22
Total MNA CGU	0.70	0.68	0.70	0.59	0.59	0.22	0.43	0.11	0.64
Total MNA Comm	0.47	0.63	0.44	0.46	–	–	0.23	0.12	0.15

NH = Nursing home; CGU = convalescence geriatric unit; Comm = community group.

Table 2 shows the correlation between the total scores in the MNA with each of its sections and the nutritional indicators for each of the three groups under study. In each of the groups, all the sections of the MNA were highly correlated with the total scores (regression coefficients from 0.43 to 0.79); in general, the coefficient of correlation was more significant in the convalescence group (especially in the anthropometric and dietetic indices) than in the nursing home group (where the subjective and global assessments are highlighted), and it was less significant in the community-based group (where the global assessment was the most important).

A moderate correlation was found with ADL, measured by the Katz index. Other studies have also shown a relation between level of physical functioning and nutritional status [20, 21].

No correlation was observed between total MNA scores and serum albumin in the nursing home population, but a correlation was found in the convalescence group, although this was weak. The low correlation with the serum albumin can be explained on a clinical basis of the greater complexity of the MNA as a nutritional evaluation tool, since it also includes risk factors and dietetic assessment among its evaluation criteria. Serum albumin decreases late in chronic undernutrition owing to reduced protein intake, and it decreases very rapidly when there is an inflammatory process [22]. It is for this reason that the highest correlation was found in the CGU patients.

The relation between the MNA score and recent weight loss was significant in all three groups, and particularly in the convalescence group. The association of MNA with BMI was also significant and it was more important in the convalescent patients. This correlation was confined to the subgroup with weight loss (Table 2).

The MNA includes sections on anthropometry, evaluation of risk situations (global assessment), dietetic survey, and self-perception of health. Owing to the fact that there are several sections, the MNA has a different profile according to the population under study. The multidimensional nature of this tool makes it useful for assessing different subclasses of elderly subjects and helps the clinician to understand some of the mechanisms determining nutritional status. For this reason, it may facilitate decision taking in therapeutic programs.

Acknowledgement

We thank Núria Casas Casanovas, who was responsible for translation of the manuscript.

References

1. Rudman D, Feller AG. Protein-calorie undernutrition in the nursing home. *J Am Geriatr Soc* 1989; 37: 173–83.
2. Alix E, Constans T, Lesourd B, Ferry M. Epidémiologie de la nutrition chez les persones âgées. *La revue de Gériatrie* 1992; 17: 525–32.
3. Morley JE, Jay A. Nutritional issues in nursing home care. *Ann Intern Med* 1995; 123: 850–9.
4. Sullivan DH, Patch GA, Walls RC, Lipschitz DA. Impact of nutrition status on morbidity and mortality in a select population of geriatric rehabilitation patients. *Am J Clin Nutr* 1990; 51: 749–58.
5. Corti MC, Guralnic LM. Serum albumin levels and physical disability as a predictor of mortality in older persons. *JAMA* 1994; 272: 1036–42.
6. Ferguson RP, O'Connor P, Crabtree B, Batchelor A, Mitchell Y, Coppola D. Serum albumin and prealbumin as a predictor of clinical outcomes of hospitalized elderly nursing home residents. *J Am Geriatr Soc* 1993; 41: 545–9.
7. Sullivan DH, Walls RC, Lipschitz DA. Protein-energy undernutrition and the risk of mortality within 1 year of hospital discharge in a select population of geriatric rehabilitation patients. *Am J Clin Nutr* 1991; 53: 599–605.
8. Moreiras O, Carbajal A, Perea I, Varela-Moreiras G, Ruiz Roso B. Nutrición y salud de las personas de edad avanzada en Europa: Euronut-Seneca. Estudio en España. *Rev Esp Geriatr Gerontol* 1993; 28: 197–242.
9. Reuben DB, Greendale GA, Harrison G. Nutrition screening in older persons. *J Am Geriatr Soc* 1995; 43: 415–25.
10. Infante Miranda F. Valoración del estado de nutrición. *Rev Clín Esp* 1994; 194: 692–700.
11. Santi Cano MJ, Barba Chacón A, Zamora Madaria E. Valoración del estado nutricional en el anciano. *Med Clin (Barcelona)* 1991; 96: 350–5.
12. Fogt EJ, Bell SJ, Blackburn GL. Nutrition assessment of the elderly. In: Morley JE, Glick Z, Rubenstein L, eds. *Geriatric nutrition. A comprehensive review,* vol 5. New York: Raven Press, 1995: 51–62.
13. Guigoz Y, Vellas B, Garry PJ. Mini Nutritional Assessment: a practical assessment tool for grading the nutritional state of elderly patients. In: *Facts and reseach in gerontology,* suppl 2. Paris: Serdi PC, 1994: 15–59.
14. Salvà A, Bolibar I, Muñoz M, Sacristan V. Un nuevo instrumento para la valoración en Geriatría: el "Mini Nutritional Assessment" (MNA). *Rev Gerontol* 1996; 6: 319–28.
15. Katz S, Ford AB, Moskowitz RW, Jackson BA, Jaffee MV. Studies of illness in the aged. The index of ADL: a standardized measure of biological and psychosocial function. *JAMA* 1963: 185: 914–9.
16. Pfeiffer EA. Short portable mental status questionaire for the assessment of organic deficit in the elderly. *J Am Geriatr Soc* 1975; 23: 433–41.

17. Salvà A, Aloy J, Castro D, *et al.* La evaluación geriátrica en una unidad de convalecencia. Análisis descriptivo de la actividad de un año. *Rev Esp Geriatr Gerontol* 1996; 31: 205–10.
18. Pertoldi W, Fragiacomo C, Rapin CH, Guigoz Y, Quadri P. The Mini Nutritional Assessment as predictor of hospital costs in geriatric patients [abstr]. *J Am Geriatr Soc* 1996; 44: 230.
19. Guigoz Y, Nourhashemi F, Vellas B. The MNA (Mini Nutritional Assessment): update. *Facts, research and intervention in geriatrics,* Serdi PC, Paris, suppl, 3rd ed. 1997: 105–12.
20. Morales Rodríguez P, González Reimers E, Santolaria Fernández F, Batista López N, Gonzalez Reyes A. Functional decline and nutritional status in a hospitalized geriatric population: sequential study. *Nutrition* 1990; 6: 469–73.
21. Galanos AN, Pieper FC, Cornoni-Huntley JC, Wales CW, Fillenbaum GG. Nutrition and function: is there a relationship between body mass index and the functional capabilities of community-dwelling elderly? *J Am Geriatr Soc* 1994; 42: 368–73.
22. Martín GM, Canalejo E. Valoración nutricional. Requerimientos calóricos y de nutrientes. *Rev Clín Esp* 1994; 194: 739–45.

Discussion

Dr. Guesry: My question regards the agreement between the same variables measured by two different observers. Of course I can easily understand why you have differences with subjective variables, depending on how you ask the question. I was pleased to see that what we discussed yesterday proved to be true in your experience. But I have difficulty in understanding why you found such a discrepancy between two observers when measuring brachial circumference. Do you have any explanation for that?

Dr. Salvá: We were surprised at these results as well. In a recent publication on the reliability of MNA, we saw similar results with respect to brachial circumference [1]. I don't know why this should be. Maybe our technique was at fault, but the nurses were trained in anthropometric techniques by the same person. Maybe someone else can offer an explanation?

Dr. Guesry: I think this is quite important, because it raises questions about the reliability of such measurements, especially for the arm. My last question to Dr. Salvá is about your measurements of MNA in 1995 and 1996 in your group of malnourished patients. You saw no improvement, though there were apparently improvements in BMI and brachial circumference. Do you have a program of nutritional support?

Dr. Salvá: First, the malnourished group is only five people. It is difficult to compare the changes in this group. Secondly, in this nursing home, the management of the patients was that normally provided by the home. We went there only to administer the MNA, and after a year and a half we returned to do the MNA again. The professionals in this nursing home had the MNA results and could institute a different nutritional regimen, but we were not responsible for that. As I said before, we have the data but we haven't analyzed them yet.

Dr. Chumlea: In relation to what Dr. Guesry was saying about the anthropometric tests: a kappa test is a nonparametric test and is probably not the most appropriate measure of reliability for the body measurements. That would be a repeated measures test.

Dr. Morley: I have a question about the length of stay. Your average of 15 days would be a very long time indeed in the USA. Even 6 days is now almost unacceptable! Was this just a subgroup that you were looking at, or is that a normal length of stay in French hospitals?

Dr. Salvá: For elderly patients, this is a normal length of stay.

Dr. Rubenstein: In one of your slides you showed a comparison of before and after for the different at-risk categories. In one of them, about 15% of people who were at risk at time 1 had their status improved by time 2. It seems quite dramatic to me that you were able to improve 15% of the group. Is a 15% improvement in the at-risk category about what you would expect? Also I'm curious about the intervention. What did you do to these people who you found to be at risk? Did you involve them in an intervention or was this just natural history?

Dr. Salvá: Of course we need to know what happened to these groups during those 18 months. We need to know who were the patients who improved and who were the ones whose nutritional status became worse? We also need to know whether the doctor in this nursing home tried to apply a treatment or nutrition plan. As I said before, we have these data, but we have not analyzed them yet.

Dr. Vellas: We need to remember that this study by Dr. Salvá was not an interventional study, only a descriptive one. I am not even sure that the physician in the nursing home knew about the MNA during the first year.

Dr. Salvá: Yes, he knew the MNA results. He had the MNA results in the clinical history. I'm not sure whether he looked at them, but he had them!

Reference

1. Gazzotti C, Pepinter A, Petermans J, Albert A. Interobserver agreement on MNA Nutritional scale of hospitalized elderly patients. *Nutr Health Aging* 1997; 1: 23–7.

Mini Nutritional Assessment (MNA): Research and Practice in the Elderly:
B. Vellas; P.J. Garry; Y. Guigoz (eds),
Nestlé Nutrition Workshop Series Clinical & Performance Programme, Vol. 1, pp. 131–140,
Nestec Ltd.; Vevey/S. Karger AG, Basel, © 1999.

MNA and Nutritional Intervention

F. Arnaud-Battandier[a], S. Lauque[b], M. Paintin[c], R. Mansourian[c], B. Vellas[b] and Y. Guigoz[c]

[a] *Nestlé Clinical Nutrition, Sèvres, France;*
[b] *Department of Internal Medicine and Clinical Gerontology, CHU Purpan-Casselardit, Toulouse, France;*
[c] *Nestlé Research Centre, Nestec Ltd., Lausanne, Switzerland*

Poor nutritional status in the elderly population is now well documented. Malnutrition affects around 20–75% of elderly patients in the hospital [1], 10–60% in nursing homes [2, 3] and 1–9% at home [4]. The causes of malnutrition are often complex and multifactorial. But whatever the cause, the clinical consequences can be serious, leading to complications of disease, poor response to drug treatment, reduced immunocompetence, and increased morbidity and mortality. Economic consequences include the increased costs associated with prolonged hospital stay and additional treatment. It is therefore important to recognize patients who are at risk of malnutrition or who are already undernourished, so that early management and corrective measures can be initiated.

There are various clinical and biochemical tools for diagnosing malnutrition, but they are not always easy to use, or else they require much clinical experience. The Mini Nutritional Assessment (MNA) was designed to detect the risk of malnutrition or malnutrition in patients [5, 6]. It is a validated tool comprising 18 easily measurable items and does not require blood testing. The MNA can be performed by health care professionals in approximately 10–15 min.

Oral supplements are a convenient way of combating malnutrition when a patient is able to take food orally. It is an acceptable option for long-term support if a variety of product categories and flavors can be offered to prevent taste fatigue and assure good compliance.

Using the MNA to evaluate the nutritional status of nursing home patients, a clinical study was performed to determine whether nutritional intervention could modify the MNA score, prevent weight loss, and possibly improve biological markers of nutritional status in patients at risk of malnutrition or already malnourished.

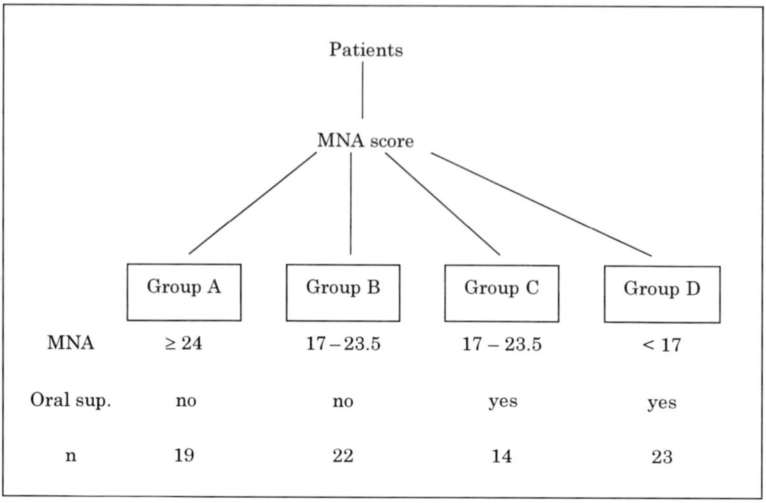

Fig. 1. Study design.

Material and Methods

Eighty-seven patients aged 67 years and over (13 men and 74 women) had an MNA performed during their stay in institutions (Toulouse area, France), and were divided into four groups according to their MNA score [5, 6]:

MNA score ≥24	Well-nourished	Group A
MNA score between 17 and 23.5	At risk of malnutrition	Groups B and C
MNA score <17	Malnourished	Group D

Groups C and D were given oral supplements.

Patients with acute pathology under chemotherapy or with compromised life expectancy were excluded, as were those with impaired intestinal digestion or absorption.

The study design (Fig. 1) was a prospective, open, controlled and randomized clinical trial (groups B and C). It was approved by the local ethics committee, conducted according to the Helsinki II declaration, and written informed consent was obtained from all subjects or their legal guardians.

The study period lasted 60 days. Dietary intakes (3-day diary), anthropometry, MNA, and biological measurements were performed at the start (day 0) and at the end of the study (day 60), while dietary intakes and body weight were also recorded at mid study (day 30). The quantity of oral supplements consumed and the choices made by the patients were recorded daily. The study lasted from December 1995 to May 1997.

Table 1. Mean total energy daily intakes (kcal/day ± SEM) at day 0 and day 60 for the 4 groups of patients

	Patient groups			
	A	B	C	D
Beginning of study (day 0)	1,689±64	1,584±60	1,558±75	1,489±59
End of study (day 60)	1,632±72	1,562±66	1,764±117	1,889±100
Supplement intakes			+393±25	+430±19

Supplement intakes corresponded to the mean daily energy ingested as supplement. p values: day 0 $p = 0.209$; day 60 $p = 0.015$; supplement intakes $p = 0.121$.

Four products specifically designed for oral nutritional supplementation were offered to the patients in groups C and D. Each of these products was offered in three flavors. They were sweet or savory, liquid or creamy products enriched with proteins, vitamins, and minerals (Tonexis® HP, Emelis®, Printania®, and Orastel®, Nestlé Clinical Nutrition, Sèvres, France; see appendix). Three supplements were offered daily to each patient, Printania being offered on odd days and Tonexis HP on even days, allowing an additional energy intake of 300–500 kcal/day. All patients were encouraged to eat their normal diet *at libitum*.

Data analysis was performed using the Number Cruncher Statistical Systems software (NCSS, Kaysville, Utah, USA). The influence of single independent factors and the analysis of the data was performed with classic one-way analysis of variance (ANOVA). Probability (p) values are given with correction by Kruskal-Wallis one-way ANOVA on ranks.

Results

Patients

Of the 87 patients recruited, 78 completed the study (males 11; females 67). Four patients died (all in group D), five were excluded for noncompliance and/or admission to hospital (group C). Age was between 67 and 98 years. There were 19 patients in group A, 22 in group B, 14 in group C, and 23 in group D.

Nutritional Intake

Daily nutritional intakes in groups A and B were very similar at day 0 and day 60 (Table 1). In group C the mean total daily energy intake increased from 1,558 to 1,815 kcal, with a decrease in spontaneous intake, the oral supplementation representing a mean intake of 393 kcal/day. In group D the total energy intake

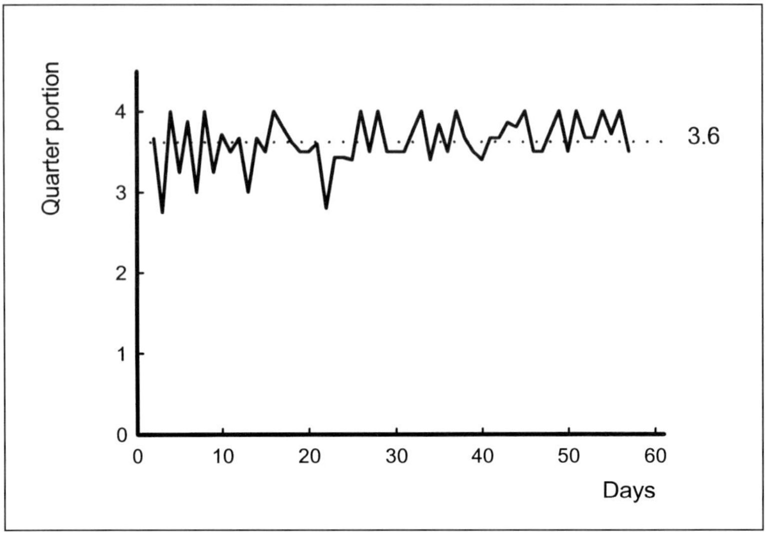

Fig. 2. Printania® compliance in group C patients from day 0 to day 60: mean daily intake (4 quarters = 1 portion = 200 ml). Dotted line = general mean (3.6 ± 0.7 quarter portions = 180 ± 35 ml; mean ± SD).

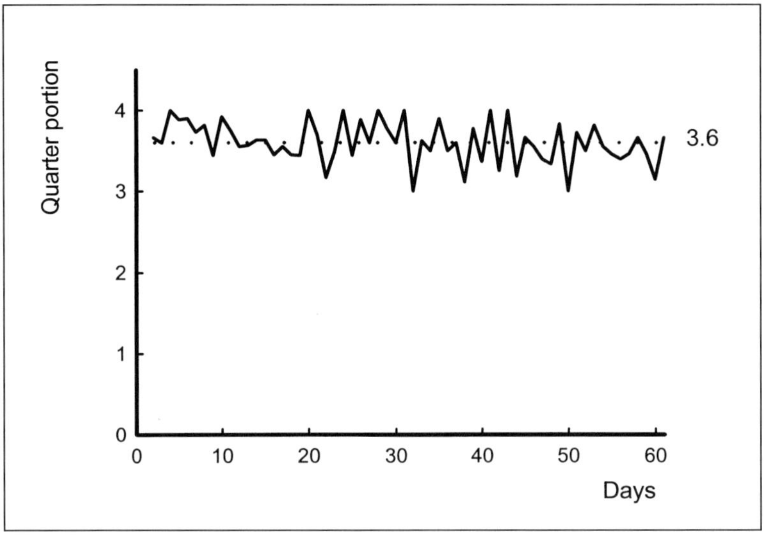

Fig. 3. Printania® compliance in group D patients from day 0 to day 60: mean daily intake (4 quarters = 1 portion = 200 ml). Dotted line = general mean (3.6 ± 0.8 quarter portions = 180 ± 38 ml; mean ± SD).

Table 2. Evolution of the MNA scores between day 0 and day 60 for the 4 groups of patients

Group	Day	MNA score			
		mean	SEM	minimum	maximum
A	0	26.1	0.5	24	28
	60	24.4	0.9	7.5	28
B	0	19.9	0.4	17	23
	60	20.6	0.8	16	24.5
C	0	19.3	0.6	17.5	22.5
	60	19.1	1.0	11.5	25
D	0	13.9	0.4	8.5	16.5
	60	17.1	0.8	6.5	23

increased from 1,489 to 1,877 kcal, but without a decrease in spontaneous intake, the oral supplementation representing a mean intake of 430 kcal/day (Table 1).

Results expressed as kcal/kg body weight/day at day 0 and day 60 showed that in groups A and B there was almost no difference in intake (29 ± 1.5 to 27 ± 1.8 kcal/kg/day, and 31 ± 1.4 to 31 ± 1.7 kcal/kg/day, respectively). On the other hand, patients in group C increased their intake from 29 ± 1.7 to 34 ± 2.0 kcal/kg/day, and in group D from 34 ± 1.3 to 43 ± 1.6 kcal/kg/day.

Compliance

Daily energy intakes remained stable during the whole study period in groups C and D, with mean daily supplement intakes of 393 ± 25 kcal/day and 430 ± 19 kcal/day, respectively ($p = 0.12$).

Analysis of product preference showed a slight decrease in intake of Emelis and Orastel in group D, but not in the other group, by the end of the study (that is, after 50 days; data not shown). These two products were offered daily, whereas Printania and Tonexis were offered on alternate days. For these latter two products, intakes remained constant during the two-month period with no taste fatigue, and total daily energy intakes from supplements remained stable over the study period (for Printania data, see Figs. 2 and 3). These results suggest that it is important to vary the taste and texture of nutritional supplements.

MNA Scores

As can be seen in Table 2, the mean MNA score did not change significantly in groups A, B, and C; however, there was a significant increase in the mean score from 13.9 to 17.1 in group D. The final MNA scores of three subjects in group A decreased <24 and one <17 (acute infection at day 45). In four patients in group C the final MNA score fell <17, but these four patients had severe pathological

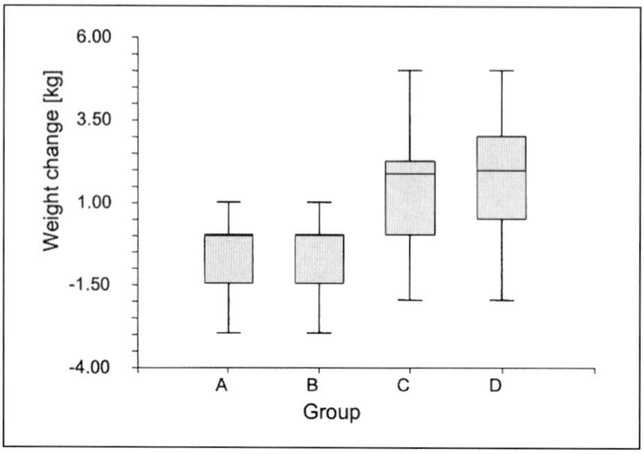

Fig. 4. Box plot of weight change between day 0 and day 60 in the four groups of patients. Box represents 50% of the population with the median and maximum gain and loss values ($p < 0.0001$).

events during the 60 days of the study (pulmonary infection, pressure sores, falls). Fifteen subjects from group D increased their final MNA score >17.

Weight Changes

As can be seen in Figure 4, there was almost no change in the median weight during the 60 days of the study in groups A and B; maximum gain and loss ranged from +1 kg to –3 kg in both.

Group C showed an increase in weight with a median of +1.5 kg, a maximum gain of +5 kg, and a maximum loss of –2 kg.

Group D showed an increase in weight with a median of +2 kg, a maximum gain of +5 kg, and a maximum loss of –2 kg.

Biological Markers

Mean values of biological markers of nutrition (albumin, prealbumin, hematocrit, hemoglobin) and inflammation (α-glycoprotein, C-reactive protein) were not altered or modified during the time course of the study (data not shown).

Discussion

Using the MNA – a validated tool for nutritional assessment – it was possible to distinguish between individuals in nursing home populations who were at risk of malnutrition, malnourished, or well-nourished. A comparative, controlled, randomized study was performed in elderly patients at risk of malnutrition subdivided in two groups, one receiving a standard diet plus an oral supplement, the other a standard diet only. For ethical reasons, malnourished patients were all supplemented with oral products.

Compliance for the oral products was satisfactory during the 60-day period of the study. It is worth noting that the at-risk supplemented population increased their total energy intake in comparison with the nonsupplemented group and in comparison with their energy intake at entry to the study. This energy increase was accompanied by a slight reduction in their spontaneous food intake. On the other hand malnourished patients were able to maintain their spontaneous energy intake at the same levels during the whole study, with oral supplementation providing additional energy. Final energy intake was significantly higher in the malnourished group than in the at-risk population.

Previous studies in elderly patients have shown that oral supplementation can be beneficial by increasing energy intake without reducing spontaneous intake [7], and have even demonstrated an improvement rather than a loss of appetite with supplementation [8].

Oral supplementation is the most appropriate way of increasing energy intake whenever possible. Its efficiency is considered equivalent to enteral nutrition given by tube [9]. However, when oral nutrition is not feasible, enteral nutrition is preferable to parenteral nutrition [10], thus maintaining gut function and the gut immune barrier.

Compliance can be maintained for long periods of time with oral supplements provided that patients are offered a wide variety of flavors, textures, tastes, smells, and colors – as we showed in this study, where consumption of oral supplements was maintained during the whole period.

Improvements in both weight and MNA reflected the increase in energy intake. With improved nutritional status, a decrease in morbidity and mortality can be expected [11]. There is a significant relation between a low MNA and increased mortality [12].

A decrease in morbidity has been clearly demonstrated in elderly patients with hip fractures given dietary supplements [13], and in the postoperative period after moderate or major gastrointestinal surgery [8]. Weight gain and improved anthropometric indices have also been reported in demented patients given supplements [14].

Conclusion

Nutritional supplements significantly increased nutrient delivery and allowed weight gain in the majority of malnourished patients and in many patients at risk of malnutrition.

Improvement in MNA scores during our study suggested that the MNA can be used as a follow-up tool in nutritional interventions.

Appendix

Names of the products used in this study were modified as follows:

Tonexis HP	⟶	Clinutren HP
Emelis	⟶	Clinutren Dessert
Printania	⟶	Clinutren Fruit
Orastel	⟶	Clinutren Soup

References

1. McWhirter JP, Pennington CR. Incidence and recognition of malnutrition in hospital. *BMJ* 1994; 308: 945–8.
2. Rudman D, Feller AG. Protein-calorie undernutrition in the nursing home. *J Am Geriatr Soc* 1989; 37: 173–83.
3. Kerstetter JE, Holhausen BA, Fitz PA. Malnutrition in the institutionalized older adult. *J Am Diet Assoc* 1992; 92: 1109–16.
4. Edington J, Kon P, Martyn CN. Prevalence of malnutrition in patients in general practice. *Clin Nutr* 1996; 15: 60–3.
5. Guigoz Y, Vellas BJ, Garry PJ. Mini Nutritional Assessment: a practical assessment tool for grading the nutritional state of elderly patients. *Facts Res Gerontol* 1994; 4 (suppl 2): 15–59.
6. Guigoz Y, Vellas B, Garry PJ. Assessing the nutritional status of the elderly: the Mini Nutritional Assessment as part of the geriatric evaluation. *Nutr Rev* 1996; 54: S59–65
7. Gray-Donald K, Payette H, Boutier V, Page S. Evaluation of the dietary intake of homebound elderly and the feasibility of dietary supplementation. *J Am Coll Nutr* 1994; 13: 277–84.
8. Rana SK, Bray J, Menzies-Gow, *et al.* Short term benefits of postoperative oral dietary supplements in surgical patients. *Clin Nutr* 1992; 11: 337–44.
9. McWhirter JP, Pennington CR. A comparison between oral and nasogastric nutritional supplements in malnourished patients. *Nutrition* 1996; 12: 502–6.
10. Hébuterne X, Broussard JF, Rampal P. Acute renutrition by cyclic enteral nutrition in elderly and younger patients. *JAMA* 1995; 273: 638–43.
11. Larsson J, Unosson M, Ek AC, *et al.* Effect of dietary supplement on nutritional status and clinical outcome in 501 geriatric patients – a randomised study. *Clin Nutr* 1990; 9: 179–84.
12. Guigoz Y, Vellas B. Test d'évaluation de l'état nutritionnel de la personne âgée: le Mini Nutritional Assessment (MNA). *Med Hyg* 1995; 53: 1965–8.
13. Delmi M, Rapin CH, Bengoa JM, *et al.* Dietary supplementation in elderly patients with fractured neck of femur. *Lancet* 1990; 335: 1013–6.
14. Carver AD, Dobson AM. Effects of dietary supplementation of elderly demented hospital residents. *J Hum Nutr Diet* 1995; 8: 389–94.

Discussion

Dr. Morley: The results were disappointing in the intervention trial, for all of us who believe in nutritional intervention. Could you speculate on why this might be?

Dr. Arnaud-Battandier: Why do you say that they are disappointing? In the group who received the supplementation, for example group D (the malnourished patients), we saw an increase in body weight and in the MNA score.

Dr. Morley: But you failed to see changes in any of the other variables that you measured, and you did not mention immune function.

Dr. Arnaud-Battandier: It is true I did not mention immune function, which was the other arm of the study. I just gave a global result. We now have to examine the values in detail and to try to gain a better understanding of the individual patients.

Dr. Morley: What I'm getting at is whether for a borderline malnourished population – these were not severely malnourished individuals – a longer time period is essential when you do design intervention studies before you start to see some of the other changes occurring.

Dr. Arnaud-Battandier: When you look at published reports, the studies usually last for 3 months. We did a 2-month study. Maybe if we had made it 1 month longer, the results would have been different.

Dr. Guigoz: When we looked at the biological variables, they were not at the level you would expect in malnutrition. We had only two patients with an albumin concentration of 30 g/l, and we had very few patients with a high CRP indicating an inflammatory process. It seems that we are detecting malnutrition, or the risk of malnutrition, before the conventional clinical indices become positive. I think that is an important point. In relation to weight change, it seemed that the other groups were still losing weight – that is, they were on the down side – but with supplementation we stopped the weight loss.

Dr. Oster: I was glad to see Dr. Arnaud-Battandier's results, because I know how difficult it is to get supplements into the patient. In our hands, in hospital we get about 200 additional kcal into the patient, with the result that the normal weight loss which occurs in geriatric patients can be stopped. They do not gain weight, but they do not lose weight either. We did an additional study where we supplemented patients for 6 months after discharge from hospital, and in the whole group there was no effect, but when we took compliance into account (users of the supplement *vs.* non-users), we saw a slight increase in ADL after 6 months of supplementation – not too convincing, but at least not a decrease.

Dr. Vellas: We need to remember that the main aim of the study was to find out whether it is possible to increase energy intake by oral supplementation. We found that in people with a low MNA score or in people at risk of malnutrition it was indeed possible to increase energy intake significantly. We shouldn't forget, however, that we had a very good dietician in Sylvie Lauque.

Dr. Rubenstein: I would like to bring that point home. I thought Dr. Arnaud-Battandier's study was very positive. Using this kind of study as a pilot, you can go on to get a big grant for a multiyear interventional study. Basically you showed that it is possible to increase intake, and you've also translated that into weight gain, and people apparently enjoyed getting the supplement. With 21 individuals in one group and 17 in the other in a 2-month follow-up period you cannot expect any other significant outcome benefit in that time. The sample size was just not designed for that.

Dr. Arnaud-Battandier: Exactly. The sample size was small because we did the immunological studies at the same time, and it was impossible to do more patients.

Dr. Morley: Did they get the supplement with the food, before the food, or in between?

Ms. Lauque: The soup was given during the meal, instead of the nursing home soup. The cream was given at the end of the meal, as a supplement to the nursing home dessert. The fruit drink was given instead of water or the regular drink. This was the usual schedule, but sometimes it varied according to the patients. Some patients preferred to have two soups and no cream, for example.

Dr. Guesry: I suggest that you should measure the time spent by the team – the nurse, the dietician and all the health workers in the different groups. We did a study 2 years ago in the biggest center for tetraplegics in France. Only by increasing the time that the nursing team spent with each patient was it possible to increase the energy consumption, well-being and physical performance. So I wonder if here there is not a certain bias between the groups in your study; obviously, when you provide a supplement, you have to spend some time with the patient. You don't just throw it on the table and leave.

Dr. Camilla: Your results seem to support the short form of the evaluation, because you only showed us results for weight and body mass index. I would like to know whether you can give us any information on protein intake as opposed to energy?

Dr. Arnaud-Battandier: I don't have the results of the protein intake measurements with me. We looked at it, and there is an increase in protein intake for group C and group D.

Dr. Guigoz: The results parallel the energy intake, because the protein energy in the supplement remained constant throughout the study. The protein intake was significantly increased in the supplemented groups.

Dr. Morley: What percentage of the food is protein in the supplements, do you know?

Dr. Guigoz: It varied from one product to another, but it was around 25%.

Dr. Miller: I want to return to a comment that Dr. Vellas made with regard to Dr. Rubenstein's scale, differentiating healthy individuals, in whom a short form might work well, from the more frail, where a more complete scale would be appropriate. I wonder whether the short form might also be useful in bringing our general practitioners – in the broad sense of that term – into our total scheme. I would want our geriatric fellows to use the whole scale and learn how to apply it to nutritional interventions and so forth. But I personally would be delighted if our general medicine residents, general internists and family practitioners would use the short form as a screen and then bring us or dieticians in to do the more complete scale and start designing the interventions. I am really excited about that possibility.

Dr. Vellas: That is one way to work. But I am concerned that a nutritional screening initiative in a nursing home or in elderly people in hospital will show nearly 100% of the population at risk. If the short form works like that, it is not useful for frail elderly people.

Dr. Morley: The nutritional screening initiative is meant to be self-scored and to encourage people to go to a doctor or ideally to a dietician to ask questions. It was developed originally to try to increase supplement use and it was coupled with a series of advertisements on TV in the United States on how every older person should be taking supplements. It was set up to be overinclusive and I agree that the advantage of what we are bearing here, even the short form for the MNA, is that it is not overinclusive.

Mini Nutritional Assessment (MNA): Research and Practice in the Elderly:
B. Vellas; P.J. Garry; Y. Guigoz (eds),
Nestlé Nutrition Workshop Series Clinical & Performance Programme, Vol. 1, pp. 141–148,
Nestec Ltd.; Vevey/S. Karger AG, Basel, © 1999.

MNA and Cost of Care

P. Quadri[a], C. Fragiacomo[b], W. Pertoldi[a], Y. Guigoz[c], F. Herrmann[d] and Ch.H. Rapin[d]

[a] *Geriatric Department, Hospital Beata Vergine, Mendrisio;*
[b] *Center for Metabolic Disease, Hospital Beata Vergine, Mendrisio;*
[c] *Nestlé Research Center, Nestec Ltd., Lausanne, Switzerland;*
[d] *Geriatric Department, HUG, Geneva, Switzerland*

Protein-energy malnutrition in elderly people living at home is observed in 5–8% of the population, whereas in subjects staying in hospitals or in other institutions, the rate varies between 30% and 60% [1–10]. It has been clearly shown that there are important clinical consequences of diminished nutritional status (increased morbidity and mortality) [11–20], as well as social repercussions (for example, a longer stay in hospital) [15–21].

Although this problem was emphasized in the past, and in spite of the proven benefits of an active nutritional support program for elderly inpatients in medical and surgical hospital wards, malnutrition in the elderly is still often underestimated [22, 23]. The difficulty in the systematic evaluation of nutritional status in elderly people is mainly caused by the impossibility of defining a single variable that is sufficiently specific and sensitive to screen for malnutrition [24]. Thus we need different anthropometric, clinical, and biological indices. Some of these have been integrated into instruments for the early evaluation of risk factors (Scale Determine, Meals On Wheels) but some still rely on laboratory tests [25–27].The value of quick and simple tests (mini-mental state, geriatric depression scale, balance scale, etc.) [28–30] in the functional examination and treatment of elderly patients has been shown by a decrease in mortality and an improvement in the quality of life and in the cost/benefit ratio [31].

Mini Nutritional Assessment (MNA) is a quick and simple screening test for elderly people that does not require laboratory tests. Validation studies have shown that the assessment score is correlated with clinical, anthropometric, and biological variables [32].

Aim of the Study

The aim of this study was to evaluate the incidence of malnutrition in elderly patients who were presumed to be well nourished, and to test for the possible relation between malnutrition and the cost and length of stay in hospital. We also wanted to identify which nutritional indices were the most sensitive in forecasting the risk of high costs and prolonged stay in hospital.

Material and Methods

We studied 166 patients, 70 years old or more, who were admitted consecutively to the Geriatric Medicine Department of the Hospital Beata Vergine in Mendrisio, Switzerland, over a 9-month period between September 1994 and May 1995.

All terminally ill subjects and those who had been in the emergency room for more than 48 h or had diseases likely to cause malnutrition (gastrointestinal disease, renal disease, malignant disease) were excluded from the study. No patients had dieted before they were recruited to the study.

In the first 72 h after hospital admission, plasma concentrations of albumin and prealbumin (thyroxin-binding protein) were determined by the nephelometric method (Behring, Marburg, Germany) in all patients, and weight, height, body mass index (BMI), and MNA (in Italian translation) were evaluated. Anthropometric measurements were performed following standard procedures [33–36].

The hospital costs were calculated by overall price × days of hospital admission + diagnostic and therapeutic services costs during admission without any drug treatment.

Statistical Analysis

Comparison of means was made using analysis of variance, while comparisons of proportions were performed by χ^2 tests. Multiple regression analyses were computed to search for predictors of costs and length of stay among components of the MNA.

Results

Table 1 shows the mean values for the various nutritional indices assessed in all subjects and in the male and female subgroups. More females than males were enrolled in the study. No significant differences between mean values of BMI, albumin, prealbumin, or MNA were found between males and females.

Table 1. Results of nutritional measurements in all patients (mean value ± SD)

	Females (n = 103)	Males (n = 63)	Total (n = 166)
Age, years	81.53±6.10	80.42±5.59	81.11±5.93
Weight, kg	60.65±13.60	69.34±12.49	63.95±13.84
Height, cm	155.13±7.30	168.65±6.70	160.26±9.65
BMI, kg/m^2	25.17±5.37	24.32±4.0	24.85±4.91
Albumin, g/l	38.16±6.04	37.18±4.42	37.79±5.63
Prealbumin, g/l	0.20±0.05	0.21±0.07	0.21±0.06
MNA, points	23.01±4.5	22.59±5.55	22.85±5.21
Cost, USD	8,839±5,219	7,533±4,377	8,344±4,957
Length of stay, days	19.75±12.90	15.61±9.27	18.18±11.83

BMI = Body mass index.

Results of the nutritional evaluations in 166 patients (as percentage of abnormal values) are given in Table 2. The proportion of patients with signs of malnutrition varied depending on the nutritional variable examined, with average values between 11% and 40 %. Our results show that MNA can assess nutritional status in elderly patients. Nutritional screening assessed by MNA classified 15% of subjects as malnourished (n = 25), 32.5% as at risk of malnutrition (n = 54), and 52.5% as well-nourished (n = 87; Fig. 1).

Descriptive analysis showed that MNA and albumin were the variables most strongly associated with cost of care and length of hospital of stay (Table 3). The cost of care and length of stay were considered in three groups of patients with different MNA scores (Table 4). There was a significant gradient in hospital admission cost according to MNA category (p = 0.0019, ANOVA). Elderly patients with a low MNA score (<17) cost significantly more than patients with an MNA of ≥24 (p = 0.002, Bonferroni), and the difference between the MNA 17–23.5 and ≥24 groups was statistically significant (p = 0.043).

There was a significant gradient in length of hospital stay according to MNA category (p = 0.0001, ANOVA). Elderly patients with a low MNA (<17) stayed significantly longer than patients with an MNA of ≥24 (p = 0.001, Bonferroni); a significant difference was also found between the 17–23.5 and ≥24 MNA groups (p = 0.018, Bonferroni).

Cost variation in relation to indices measured at the time of hospital admission (weight, height, albumin, prealbumin, BMI, MNA, C-reactive protein, sex, age) was examined in a multiple regression model. MNA alone explained 6.6% of the total variance of cost (R^2); adding age and sex improved this to 8.7%, and adding albumin and C-reactive protein improved it further to 14.4%. Using mul-

Table 2. Results of nutritional evaluation: % abnormal values in 166 patients

	Patients n	%
Weight loss > 3 kg	19	11
MNA < 17 points	25	15
Albumin < 35 g/l	50	30
Albumin < 30 g/l	10	6
BMI < 23 kg/m^2	52	31
BMI < 20 kg/m^2	23	13
Prealbumin < 0.20 g/l	67	40

BMI = Body mass index.

Table 3. Cost of care and hospital length of stay in group A (well-nourished) and group B (malnourished)

	Costs, USD	*p*	Length of stay, days	*p*
Group A				
MNA ⩾ 24	7,299		14.5	
BMI ⩾ 23	8,114		17.0	
Albumin ⩾ 35 g/l	7,707		16.5	
Prealbumin ⩾ 0.2 g/l	7,726		17.0	
Group B				
MNA < 17	11,173	0.0010	26	0.00001
BMI < 23	8,844	0.382	20	0.1381
Albumin < 35 g/l	9,818	0.0117	22	0.0084
Prealbumin < 0.2 g/l	9,524	0.0518	20	0.1341

Table 4. MNA, length of stay, and hospital cost (mean ± SD; n = 166 patients)

MNA score	n	Days	USD
< 17	25	26 ± 3.0^{a}	$11{,}173 \pm 1{,}322^{c}$
17–23.5	54	20 ± 1.5^{b}	$9{,}112 \pm 613^{d}$
≥ 24	87	$15 \pm 1.1^{a,b}$	$7{,}299 \pm 517^{c,d}$

^{a} $p < 0.001$; ^{b} $p < 0.018$; ^{c} $p < 0.002$; ^{d} $p < 0.043$.

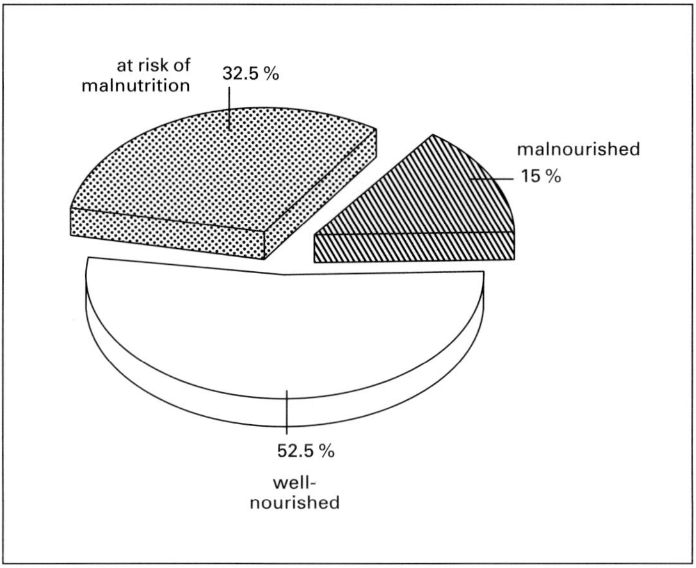

Fig. 1. Nutritional screening by MNA in 166 patients.

tiple regression analysis to search for predictors of cost among components of the MNA, we found none that were significantly associated, even though the model explained 19.2% of the cost variance.

MNA alone explained 11.0% of the total variance of length of stay (R^2); adding age and sex improve this to 14.5%, and adding albumin and C-reactive protein improved it further to 19.5%. Using multiple regression analysis to search for predictors of length of stay among components of the MNA, we found none that were significantly associated, even though the model explained 24.4% of variance of length of stay.

Conclusions

In elderly patients in hospital, who were assumed to be well-nourished, the prevalence of malnutrition in fact varied between 10% and 40% according to the nutritional index evaluated. Great variability in cost of care and length of hospital stay was observed; nevertheless these variables consistently increased in line with deterioration in nutritional status.

The cost and length of hospital stay were inversely correlated with plasma albumin concentration. Plasma albumin, both on admission and during the course of hospital treatment, is a predictor of morbidity, mortality, and length of stay [37–39].

An MNA score of <17 is associated with a higher cost of care and a longer hospital stay. The MNA represents a simple and inexpensive form of nutritional assessment capable of predicting increased cost of care and prolonged stay in hospital. Attention to nutritional status in old people improves health status and quality of life [40–45].

These preliminary results show the importance of evaluating and attending to nutritional status in old people, thereby improving their health and quality of life and reducing health costs. Early screening of nutritional status using MNA in conjunction with a nutritional intervention program could help reduce health care costs in geriatric medicine.

References

1. Albiin N, Asplund K, Bjermer L. Nutritional status of medical patients on emergency admission to hospital. *Acta Med Scand* 1982; 212: 151–6.
2. Constans T, Bacq Y, Brechot J-F, Guilmot J-L, Choutet P, Lamisse F. Protein-energy malnutrition in elderly medical patients. *J Am Geriatr Soc* 1992; 40: 263–8.
3. Hill G, Pickford I, Young G. Malnutrition in surgical patients. An unrecognised problem. *Lancet* 1977; i: 689–92.
4. O'Leary JP, Dunn GD, Basil S, Butler B, Long S, Nichols A, Waller R. Incidence of malnutrition among patients admitted to a VA hospital. *South Med J* 1982; 75: 1095–8.
5. Bienia R, Ratcliff S, Barbour GL, Kummer M. Malnutrition in the hospitalized geriatric patient. *J Am Geriatr Soc* 1982; 30: 433–6.
6. Pinchovsky-Devin GD, Kaminski MV. Incidence of protein caloric malnutrition in the nursing home population. *J Am Coll Nutr* 1987; 6: 109–12.
7. Shaver HJ, Loper JA, Lutes RA. Nutritional status of nursing home patients. *J Parenter Enter Nutr* 1980; 4: 367–70.
8. Henderson CT. Nutrition and malnutrition in the elderly nursing home patient. *Clin Geriatr Med* 1988; 4: 527–47.
9. Rudman D, Feller AG. Protein calorie undernutrition in the nursing home. *J Am Geriatr Soc* 1989; 37: 173–83.
10. Euronut Seneca Investigators. Nutritional status: haematology and albumin. *Eur J Clin Nutr* 1991; 45 (S3): 43–52.
11. Fischer J, Johnson MA. Low body and weight loss in the aged. *J Am Diet Assoc* 1990; 90: 1697–706.
12. Relation of anthropometric and dynamometric variables to serious postoperative complications. *BMJ* 1980; 28: 899–901.
13. Jeejeebhoy KN. The functional basis of assessment. In: *Nutritional support: nutrition and metabolism in patient care.* Philadelphia: WB Saunders, 1988: 739–51.
14. Romagnoli-Juillard A, Rapin C-H, Poirot P. Nutrition and immunity in the elderly. In: Chandra RK, ed. *Nutrition, immunity and illness in the elderly.* New York: Pergamon Press, 1984: 143–9.
15. Herrmann FR, Safran C, Levkoff SE, Minaker KL. Serum albumin level on admission as a predictor of death, length of stay, and readmission. *Arch Intern Med* 1992; 152: 125–30.
16. Agarwal N, Acervedo F, Leighton LS, Cayten CG, Pitchumoni CS. Predictive ability of various nutritional variables for mortality in elderly people. *Am J Clin Nutr* 1988; 48: 1173–8.
17. Tayback M, Kumanyika S, Chu E. Body weight as a risk factor in the elderly. *Arch Intern Med* 1990; 150: 1065–72.
18. Rich MW, Keller AJ, Scheihtman KB, Marshall WG, Kouchoukos NT. Increased complications and prolonged hospital stay in elderly cardiac surgical patients with low albumin. *Am J Cardiol* 1989; 63: 714–18.

19. Constans T, Bacq Y, Brechot J-F, Guilmot J-L, Choutet P, Lamisse F. Protein-energy malnutrition in elderly medical patients. *J Am Geriatr Soc* 1992; 40: 263–8.
20. Sullivan DH, Walls RC, Lipschitz DA. Protein energy undernutrition and the risk of mortality within 1 year of hospital discharge in a select population of geriatric patients. *Am J Clin Nutr* 1991; 53: 599–605.
21. Weinsier RL, Hunker EM, Krumdieck CL, Butterworth CE. A prospective evaluation of general medical patients during the hospitalization. *Am J Clin Nutr* 1979; 32: 418–26.
22. Mowe M, Bhomer T. The prevalence of undiagnosed protein caloric undernutrition in a population of hospitalized elderly patients. *Am Geriatr Soc* 1991; 39: 1089–92.
23. Miller DK, Morley JE, Rubinstein LZ, *et al.* Formal geriatric instruments and the care of elderly general medical outpatients. *J Am Geriatr Soc* 1990; 38: 645–51.
24. Reuben DB, Greendale GA, Harrison GG. Nutritional screening in older persons. *J Am Coll Gerontol* 1995; 43: 415–25.
25. Millen Posner B, Jette AM, Smith KW, Miller DR. Nutrition and health risks in the elderly: the nutrition screening initiative. *Am J Public Health* 1993; 83: 972–8.
26. Dwyen JT, White JV, Ham RJ, Lipschitz DA, Wellman NS. Consensus of the nutrition screening initiative: risk factors and indications of poor nutritional status in older Americans. *J Am Diet Assoc* 1991; 91: 783–7.
27. Morley JE. Why do physicians fail to recognize and treat malnutrition in older persons? *J Am Geriatr Soc* 1991; 39: 1139–40.
28. Folstein ME, Folstein SE, High PR. Mini Mental State: a practical method for grading the cognitive state of patients for the clinician. *J Psychiatr Res* 1975; 12: 189–95.
29. Yesavage JA, Brink TL, Rose TL. Development and validation of a geriatric depression screening scale. *J Psychiatr Res* 1983; 17: 37–42.
30. Tinetti ME, Williams TF, Mayewski R. Fall risk index for elderly patients based on number of chronic disabilities. *Am J Med* 1986; 80: 429–34.
31. Stuck AE, Siu Al, Wieland DG, *et al.* Comprehensive geriatric assessment: a meta-analysis of controlled trials. *Lancet* 1993; 342: 1032–6.
32. Guygoz Y, Vellas B, Garry PJ. Mini Nutritional Assessment: a practical assessment tool for grading the nutritional state of elderly patients. *Facts Res Gerontol* 1994; suppl N2; 15–59.
33. Chumlea WC, Steinbaugh ML, Roche AF. Nutritional anthropometric assessment in elderly persons 65 to 90 years. *J Nutr Elderly* 1985; 4: 39–51.
34. Chumlea WC, Roche AF, Mukherjee D. Some anthropometric indices of body composition for elderly adults. *J Gerontol* 1986; 41: 36–9.
35. Chumlea WC, Roche AF, Mukherjee D. *Nutritional assessment in the elderly through anthropometry.* Columbus, Ohio: Ross Laboratories, 1987.
36. Lohman TG, Roche AF, Martorell R. *Anthropometric standardization reference manual.* Champaigu, Illinois: Human Kinetic Books, 1988.
37. Sullivan DH. Risk factors for early hospital readmission in a select population of geriatric rehabilitation patients: the significance of nutritional status. *J Am Geriatr Soc* 1992; 40: 792–8.
38. Bonnefoy M, Ayzac L, Bienvenu J, Boisson RC, Rys L, Jauffret M. Facteurs prédictifs du devenir immédiat de patients âgés hospitalisés à la suite d'un événement aigu. *Rev Gériatr* 1995; 20: 265–72.
39. Anderson CF, Moxness K, Meister J, Burrit MF. The sensitivity and specificity of nutrition related variables in relationship to the duration of hospital stay and the rate of complications. *Mayo Clin Proc* 1984; 59: 477–83.
40. Delmi M, Rapin C-H, Bengoa J-M, Delmas PD, Vasey J-P, Bonjour J-P. Dietary supplementation in elderly patients with fractured neck of the femur. *Lancet* 1990; 335: 1013–6.
41. Larsson J, Unosson AC, Nilsson L, Thorslund S, Bjurulf P. Effects of dietary supplement on nutritional status and clinical outcome in 501 geriatric patients. *Clin Nutr* 1990; 9: 179–84.
42. Tkatch L, Rapin C-H, Rizzoli R, *et al.* Benefits of oral protein supplementation in elderly patients with fracture of the proximal femur. *J Am Coll Nutr* 1992; 11: 519–25.
43. Dempsey DT, Mullen JL, Buzby GP. The link between nutritional status and clinical outcome: can nutritional intervention modify it? *Am J Clin Nutr* 1988; 47: 352–6.
44. Rochat T. Nutrition et maladie respiratoire: l'exemple de la broncho-pneumopathie obstructive chronique. *Méd Hyg* 1994; 52: 1128–30.
45. Chandra RK. Effect of vitamin and trace-element supplementation on immune responses and infection in elderly subjects. *Lancet* 1992: 340: 1124–7.

Discussion

Dr. Guesry: Maybe I missed the point, but did you remove the patients who died from your study, because obviously, if they died, this should shorten their length of stay and reduce the cost. So it could introduce a bias in the most severely malnourished patients. If so you have sadly reduced the power of your study.

Dr. Fragiacomo: The patients who died were not included.

Dr. Zulian: Why did you exclude patients with diseases that have an impact on nutrition? And how did you select those diseases?

Dr. Fragiacomo: We excluded all patients with chronic gastrointestinal disease or renal disease, malignant disease, metabolic disease including poorly controlled diabetes, hypo- and hyperthyroidism.

Dr. Zulian: So what was left then, after having excluded all these types of disease?

Dr. Fragiacomo: Most of the patients had cardiovascular disease (64.5%), neurologic and psychiatric disease (44.5%), respiratory (18%) or metabolic (19%) disease. A small proportion had hematological, renal, gastrointestinal or rheumatological diseases.

Mini Nutritional Assessment (MNA): Research and Practice in the Elderly:
B. Vellas; P.J. Garry; Y. Guigoz (eds),
Nestlé Nutrition Workshop Series Clinical & Performance Programme, Vol. 1, pp. 149–155,

Animal Model: Metabolic and Thermic Responses to Diet and Environment (4°C) in Obesity during Aging in the LA/Ntul//-*cp* Rat

Orien L. Tulp and Susan P. DeBolt

Drexel University, Philadelphia, Pa., USA

The aging represent the single most rapidly increasing segment of the population of Westernized countries and throughout much of the world [1, 2]. In the USA, obesity is the major nutritionally related health complication of adults and older Americans, where it has been variously reported to affect up to one in three or more of that population [3–5]. While obesity is a significant contributing risk factor in the pathophysiology of numerous metabolic diseases common in Westernized society, including non-insulin-dependent diabetes mellitus (NIDDM), hyperlipidemia, and other metabolic disorders, the precise mechanism or mechanisms through which it may contribute to an increased risk of premature morbidity and mortality have not been fully clarified [3, 4]. As nations become progressively more industrialized, the incidence of obesity and overweight conditions and their pathophysiologic sequelae have typically become increased, and along with those changes, there is a correspondingly greater dependence on the health care industry of those nations [5–8].

An animal model of aging and obesity has been developed in our laboratory in an attempt to gain insight into specific pathophysiologic mechanisms associated with aging and obesity [9]. The model shows marked obesity, impaired carbohydrate tolerance, hyperamylinemia, hypertriglyceridemia and hypercholesterolemia, and an impaired capacity for nonshivering thermogenesis (NST) and energy expenditure from an early age [9–12]. To determine the effects of obesity on metabolic and hormonal responses to aging and to the capacity for NST during aging, groups of lean and obese LA/Ntul//-*cp* rats were subjected to measurements

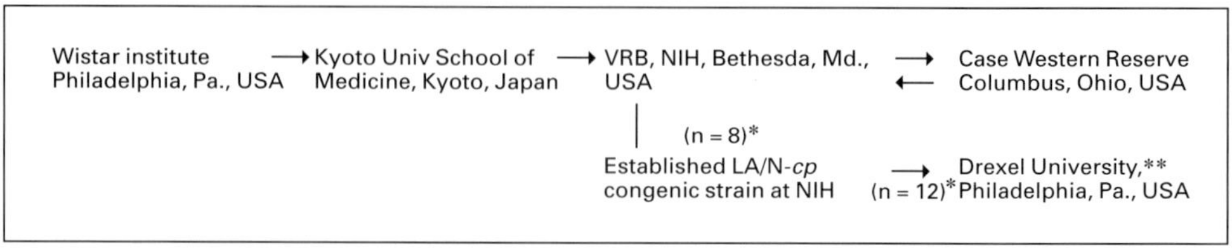

Fig. 1. Development of the LA/Ntul//-*cp* (corpulent) rat [13, 14]. * Number of backcrosses completed. ** Designated as LA/Ntul//-*cp* by ILAR.

of VO_2 in young (3–6 months), middle-aged (12–16 months), old (24–30 months), and aged (32–36 months; lean only) states under conditions of thermal neutrality (30 °C). The findings of the study indicated that aging in this unique animal model is associated with progressive declines in the normal dietary, metabolic, and hormonal responses to diet and environment, in a manner similar to that observed in man [1, 2]. Moreover, the effects of obesity further exacerbate those changes, with a corresponding negative impact on metabolic factors related to optimal health and longevity. A summary of the findings in this animal model follows below.

Development and Biometric Characteristics of the LA/Ntul//-*cp* Strain

The congenic LA/Ntul//-*cp* rat was derived from an original cross between the Koletsy rat and a congenic LA/N (Lister-Albany/NIH) strain of unknown origin at the National Institutes of Health, Bethesda, Md., USA (Fig. 1). Animals which carried the obesity (*cp*) trait were then backcrossed to the original LA/N strain until establishment of the congenic status was achieved in the new strain [13]. The animals were established in the Drexel University laboratory as the congenic LA/Ntul//-*cp* from offspring derived from the 12th backcross of the NIH strain, and are maintained in a closed environment as an SPF-VAF colony [9]. LA/Ntul//-*cp* rats from our laboratory have shown the greatest longevity of any obese rodent strain, with lean rats often surviving to over 4 years and obese rats to 30–36 months in conventional, geographically isolated housing with *ad libitum* access to rodent chow and house water [9].

The *cp* trait has also been established in other strains in a similar manner, including the SHR/Ntul//-*cp*, the WKY/N-*cp*, and others, resulting in the development of new strains with uniquely different metabolic characteristics including diabetes (NIDDM), atherosclerotic traits, renal dysfunction, and congestive heart failure [13–15]. Growth and adiposity data from LA/Ntul//-*cp* rats (Fig. 2, Table 1) show that male rats typically weigh about twice as much as similar aged

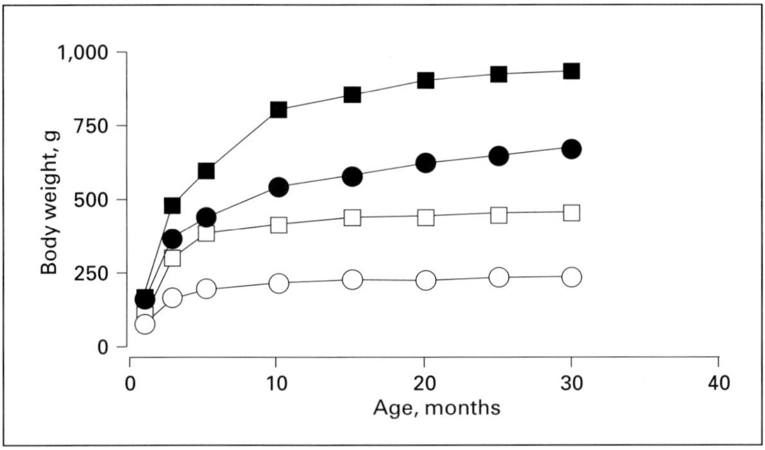

Fig. 2. Body weights of rats. Growth curves of LA/Ntul//-*cp* rats. Body weights were obtained in approximately 600 fed rats between 8 and 11 a.m., with 10–20 rats for each individual data point. □ = Lean male; ○ = lean female; ■ = obese male; ● = obese female. Body weight of obese > lean in both sexes from 1 month of age (ANOVA).

female rats in the lean phenotype, and that for any given age, weights of obese rats of either gender range between 2.5- to threefold more than normally fed lean littermates. Adiposity, computed as the sum of the dorsal and retroperitoneal fat pads over body weight (Table 1), indicates that obese female rats were substantially fatter than their lean littermates by 1–2 months of age, and that body fat content increased markedly from about the time of adolescence to adulthood, when it may represent 50% or more of the total body mass [9, 15, 16].

In normally lean animals in this and other studies, body weight became substantially stabilized by 5 months of age (Fig. 2, Table 1), with only gradual increases in body weight and energy intake (Table 1) and until 2 years of age. By 3 years of age, both energy intakes and body weights began to decline, while body fat content was preserved. In contrast, obese animals continued to gain weight and to increase in relative adiposity throughout the duration of this study, despite abundant reserves of interscapular brown adipose tissue (Table 1). The progressive increases in weight and adiposity in both phenotypes were associated with gradual decreases in energy efficiency, with the greatest efficiency observed in obese animals aged 2 years or more.

In contrast, serum thyroid hormone profiles during the same period changed markedly. Serum T3, expressed as a percentage of the serum T4 concentration, increased more than twofold in both sexes and phenotypes by 2–3 years of age – from 2.8% of the T4 concentration when 5 months of age to some 5.8% at 3 years of age in lean rats, and from 3% of the T4 at 5 months of age to over 7% of the T4

Table 1. Body weight and metabolic variables of aging rats

	Lean				Obese		
Age, months:	5	15	25	36	5	15	25
Body weight, g	224±9	247±6	263±8	235±5	444±15	608±27	746±3
Relative adiposity	1.2±0.1	1.4±0.2	1.5±0.4	1.7±03	7.6±0.1	10.1±0.4	17.5±1
Energy intake, kcal/day	53±3	55±2	58±6	44±5	84±5	114±13	106±7
Fluid intake, ml/day	23±2	28±2	35±4	n.d.	33±3	40±4	52±4
Caloric efficiency, kcal/kg BW/day	0.24±0.03	0.23±0.02	0.21±0.02	0.18±0.01	0.20±0.03	0.19±0.02	0.15±0
RMR, ml O_2/BW-0.75	13.6±0.9	14.3±0.6	12.3±0.8	11.8±0.5	12.3±0.5	10.4±0.6	10.8±0
VO_2 in cold at 45 min	24.9±2.9	25.9±1.0	23.6±1.5	14.4±0.8	21.4±1.3	15.1±0.5	14.0±0
VO_2 + NE, 100 µg/kg BW[a]	19.3±1.1	18.8±0.8	13.1±1.0	12.2±0.4	15.2±1.1	12.6±0.9	13.1±0
Serum T3	1.2±0.1	1.4±0.1	1.4±0.1	1.3±0.2	1.4±0.1	1.6±0.1	2.0±0
Serum T4	42.6±3.5	31.7±1.6	32.7±1.3	22.5±0.3	46.7±4.5	26.3±1.6	26.0±1
Fasting serum insulin, µIU/ml	30±6	35±6	22±2	n.d.	139±12	113±11	109±2
Fasting serum glucose, m*M*	5.4±0.2	4.6±0.4	5.0±0.3	n.d.	5.8±0.3	5.8±0.4	5.5±0

Data are mean ± 1 SEM, n = 10 rats/group. n.d. = Measurement not done; RMR = resting metabolic rate; NE = norepinephrine.
[a] Measures taken 30 min after injection.

content by 2 years of age in obese rats. These increases in the percent and total concentration of T3 were found to be associated with gradual decreases in T4 concentrations and in a delayed clearance *in vivo* of both thyroid hormones (T3 and T4) in the obese phenotype [17]. When the thyroidal kinetics are considered in the light of the resting metabolic rate (RMR) and energy efficiency data, the conclusions are consistent with an age-related refractoriness to thyroid hormones, particularly T3 in aging obese rats.

In other studies, the rate of T3 neogenesis from T4 in several tissues was also found to be lower in pre-obese than lean animals of this strain [18], consistent with a decreased rate of thyroidal monodeiodination in peripheral tissues, and with a gradual decrease in thyroid hormone-mediated components of energy metabolism in the obese phenotype. Impaired serum thyroxine monodeiodination was also noted in other obese, hyperinsulinemic models, including both obese-diabetic (NIDDM) SHR/Ntul//-*cp* rats [19] and obese Zucker rats [20], suggestive of a possible role for insulin resistance in mediating the impairments in thyroid hormone metabolism which were observed in this study.

Thus the results of this study are consistent with an improved economy of energy utilization and storage in association with aging, an economy that is further enhanced in the obese phenotype. Measures of resting metabolism (summarized in Table 1) reflected a gradual decline in RMR in both phenotypes, but the magnitude of the decline in energy expenditure was more pronounced in the obese than the lean phenotype. In aging LA/Ntul//-*cp* rats, the VO_2 of lean rats was greater than of obese rats, and decreased progressively in both phenotypes at each age studied (Table 1). In addition, the thermic responses to norepinephrine (100 μg NE/kg body weight, s.c.), feeding, and acute cold exposure (2–4 °C) also decreased progressively with age, such that at the oldest ages the thermic responses to variables of diet and environment were no longer statistically significant. The food and fluid intake data are consistent with a greater proportion of lipid utilization with progressive aging in both phenotypes, in concert with the age-related thyroidal responses noted above. The thermic and cold responses to carbohydrate feeding also declined with progressive aging in both phenotypes (data not shown). Fasting insulin and glucose concentrations of lean rats remained euglycemic throughout the study (Table 1), while in obese animals, the fasting insulin and the insulin to glucose ratios were markedly increased throughout the study, consistent with moderate insulin resistance and glucose intolerance of long-standing duration in the obese phenotype. Glucose uptake and incorporation into muscle glycogen was also impaired [11], and both the glucose and the insulin area following an oral glucose tolerance became increased from 2 months of age [10, 21], also indicating long-standing insulin resistance in the obese phenotype. Insulin resistance has been reported by several investigators to play a significant role in the impaired thermic responses to diet and environment in animal models [9, 15, 21–25], and is presumed to be a contributing factor in the impaired thermic responses and other chronic metabolic sequelae of the present study.

Summary

The results of this study indicate that aging is associated with progressive declines in the normal dietary and metabolic responses to diet and environment in this animal model. The normal thermic and hormonal responses to diet and environment are thought to contribute to the fine regulation of energy balance by modulation of the efficiency of energy utilization or storage [25]. In the obese phenotype, the declines in the above variables may be further complicated by the presence of long-standing insulin resistance, and by perturbations in the normal metabolism and action of thyroid hormones, particularly T3. These may further contribute, individually or in combination with other factors, to an enhancement of energy storage and thereby contribute to maintaining the obese state. Moreover, the effects of progressive increases in obesity further exacerbate the decline in the economy of energy utilization and storage. Thus the impact of these physiologic changes of aging and obesity may impart significant alterations on the efficiency of energy metabolism, which in turn may contribute to some of the pathophysiologic changes associated with longevity, and could influence nutritional indices in affected individuals. As nations become progressively more industrialized, the incidence of overweight conditions – including obesity, NIDDM, and related metabolic disorders – has been shown to become increased and, along with those changes, the metabolic and pathophysiologic sequelae related to those disorders become more common [6–8]. A greater understanding of mechanisms of impaired energy metabolism and energy balance in aging may provide new insight into the nutritional factors that may contribute to obesity in aging, their modulation, and the emergence of a longer, healthier lifestyle.

Acknowledgements

We wish to thank Ms. Jacomina Winters and Ms. Amy Parkman for contributions to manuscript preparation. Support was provided from grants-in-aid from the American Diabetes Association, the American Dietetic Association, and institutional support.

References

1. Munro HN. The challenges of research into nutrition and aging. In: Munro HN, Danford DE, eds. *Human nutrition. Volume 6. Nutrition, aging, and the elderly.* New York: Plenum, 1989: 1–2.
2. Letsou AP, Price LS. Health, aging and nutrition: an overview. *Clin Geriatric Med* 1987; 3: 253–60.
3. VanItallie TT, Abraham S. In Hirsch J, ed. *Recent advances in obesity research IV.* London: John Libbey, 1985: 1–7.
4. Kissebah AH, Freedman DS, Pairis AN. Health risks of obesity. *Med Clin North Am* 1989; 73: 111–38.
5. Kuzmarski RJ, Flegal KM, Campbell SM, Johnson CL. Increasing prevalence of overweight among US adults: the National Health and Nutrition Examination Survey 1991. *JAMA* 1994; 272: 205–11.
6. Kannel WB. Effect of weight on cardiovascular disease. *Nutrition* 1997; 13: 157–8.

7. Solomons NW, Gross R. Urban nutrition in developing countries. *Nutr Rev* 1995; 53: 90–4.
8. Gross R. Dynamics of urbanization and nutrition: a new dimension of the "forth world". *Nutrition* 1997; 13: 149–51.
9. Tulp OL. Characteristics of thermogenesis, obesity, and longevity in the LA/N-*cp* rat. *ILAR News* 1990; 32: 32–8.
10. Michaelis OE, Ellwood KC, Tulp OL, Greenwood MRC. Effect of feeding sucrose or starch diets on parameters of glucose tolerance in the LA/N-corpulent rat. *Nutr Res* 1986; 6: 95–9.
11. Huang H-JS, Young AA, Koda JE, Tulp OL, Johnson MJ, Cooper GJS. Hyperamylinemia, hyperinsulinemia, and insulin resistance in genetically obese LA/N-*cp* rats. *Hypertension* 1992; 19 [suppl I]: 101–109.
12. Abdullahi A, Tulp OL, Schnitzer-Polokof R. The effects of acarbose on cholesterolgenesis in obese and obese-diabetic rats. *Drugs in development. Volume 1. α-Glucosidase inhibitors. Potential uses in diabetes.* Vaselli J, Maggio CA, Scriabine A, eds. Neva Press, Branford, CT, USA 1993: 133–43.
13. Hansen CT. The development of the SHR/N- and LA/N-*cp* (corpulent) rat strains. In: *New models of genetically obese rats for studies in diabetes, heart disease, and complications of obesity.* (NIH publication.) Bethesda, Maryland: Division of Research Services, Veterinary Resources Branch, NIH, 1988: 7–10.
14. Greenhouse DD, Michaelis OE, McCune SA. Development of corpulent rat strains. *Frontiers in diabetes research. Lessons from animal diabetes III.* E. Shafrir, ed. Smith Gordin Publishers, London, UK 1990: 375–7.
15. Tulp OL. Thermogenesis and obesity in the LA/N-*cp* and SHR/N-*cp* rat strains. In: *New models of genetically obese rats for studies in diabetes, heart disease, and complications of obesity.* (NIH publication.) Bethesda, Maryland: Division of Research Services, Veterinary Resources Branch, NIH, 1988: 75–9.
16. Klurfeld DM, Lloyd LM, Welch CB, Davis MJ, Tulp OL, Kritchevsky D. Reduction of enhanced mammary carcinogenesis in LA/N-*cp* (corpulent) rats by energy restriction. *Proc Soc Exp Biol Med* 1991; 196: 381–4.
17. Tulp OL, Paz Nava M, DeBolt SP. Thyroidal status and glucose oxidation in aging lean and obese LA/N-*cp* rats [abstr]. *FASEB J* 1993; 7: A280.
18 Tulp OL, McKee STD. Triiodothyronine (T3) neogenesis in lean and obese LA/N-*cp* rats. *Biochem Biophys Res Commun* 1986; 140: 134–42.
19. Tulp OL, DeBolt SP, McKee SK, Michaelis OE. Adaptive thermogenesis and energy metabolism in the SHR/N-*cp* rat. In: Shafrir E, ed. *Frontiers in diabetes research. Lessons from animal diabetes III.* 1990: 381–6.
20. Young RA, Tulp OL, Horton ES. Thyroid and growth responses of young Zucker obese and lean rats to a low protein-high carbohydrate diet. *J Nutr* 1980; 14: 1421–31.
21. Tulp OL, Haugaard N, Hess ME. Metabolic responses to acarbose in the corpulent rat. In: Vaselli J, Maggio CA, Scriabine A, eds. *Drugs in development. Volume 1. α-Glucosidase inhibitors. Potential uses in diabetes.* 1993: 61–73.
22. Bukowiecki LJ, Kearney J, Collet AJ, Tulp O, Perusse F. Energy expenditure, insulin resistance, and obesity. In: Oomura Y, Tarul S, Inoae S, Shimazu T, eds. *Progress in obesity research.* London: John Libbey, 1990: 167–73.
23. Tulp OL, McKee STD, Sandler C. The role of insulin resistance on impaired energy expenditure in the LA/N-*cp* (LA-corpulent) rat [abstr]. *Proc Nutr Soc* 1988; 47: 26A.
24. Shibata H, Perusse F, Bukowiecki LJ. The role of insulin resistance in nonshivering thermogenesis. *Can J Physiol Pharmacol* 1986; 65: 152–8.
25. Himms Hagen J. Brown adipose tissue metabolism and thermogenesis. *Annu Rev Nutr* 1985; 5: 69–94.

Appendix

Nestlé CLINICAL NUTRITION

Original Version

MINI NUTRITIONAL ASSESSMENT
MNA®

ID# ____________

Last Name: ______________ First Name: ______________ M.I. _____ Sex: _____ Date: ______________

Age: _____ Weight, kg: ___________ Height, cm: ___________ Knee Height, cm: ______________

Complete the form by writing the numbers in the boxes. Add the numbers in the boxes and compare the total assessment to the Malnutrition Indicator Score.

ANTHROPOMETRIC ASSESSMENT

	Points
1. Body Mass Index (BMI) (weight in kg) / (height in m)^2 a. BMI < 19 = 0 points b. BMI 19 to < 21 = 1 point c. BMI 21 to < 23 = 2 points d. BMI ≥ 23 = 3 points	☐
2. Mid-arm circumference (MAC) in cm a. MAC < 21 = 0.0 points b. MAC 21 ≤ 22 = 0.5 points c. MAC > 22 = 1.0 points	☐.☐
3. Calf circumference (CC) in cm a. CC < 31 = 0 points b. CC ≥ 31 = 1 point	☐
4. Weight loss during last 3 months a. weight loss greater than 3kg (6.6 lbs) = 0 points b. does not know = 1 point c. weight loss between 1 and 3 kg (2.2 and 6.6 lbs) = 2 points d. no weight loss = 3 points	☐

GENERAL ASSESSMENT

5. Lives independently (not in a nursing home or hospital) a. no = 0 points b. yes = 1 point	☐
6. Takes more than 3 prescription drugs per day a. yes = 0 points b. no = 1 point	☐
7. Has suffered psychological stress or acute disease in the past 3 months a. yes = 0 points b. no = 2 points	☐
8. Mobility a. bed or chair bound = 0 points b. able to get out of bed/chair but does not go out = 1 point c. goes out = 2 points	☐
9. Neuropsychological problems a. severe dementia or depression = 0 points b. mild dementia = 1 point c. no psychological problems = 2 points	☐
10. Pressure sores or skin ulcers a. yes = 0 points b. no = 1 point	☐

DIETARY ASSESSMENT

	Points
11. How many full meals does the patient eat daily? a. 1 meal = 0 points b. 2 meals = 1 point c. 3 meals = 2 points	☐
12. Selected comsumption markers for protein intake • At least one serving of dairy products (milk, cheese, yogurt) per day? yes ☐ no ☐ • Two or more servings of legumes or eggs per week? yes ☐ no ☐ • Meat, fish or poultry every day? yes ☐ no ☐ a. if 0 or 1 yes = 0.0 points b. if 2 yes = 0.5 points c. if 3 yes = 1.0 points	☐.☐
13. Consumes two or more servings of fruits or vegetables per day? a. no = 0 points b. yes = 1 point	☐
14. Has food intake declined over the past three months due to loss of appetite, digestive problems, chewing or swallowing difficulties? a. severe loss of appetite = 0 points b. moderate loss of appetite = 1 point c. no loss of appetite = 2 points	☐
15. How much fluid (water, juice, coffee, tea, milk,...) is consumed per day? (1 cup = 8 oz.) a. less than 3 cups = 0.0 points b. 3 to 5 cups = 0.5 points c. more than 5 cups = 1.0 points	☐.☐
16. Mode of feeding a. Unable to eat without assistance = 0 points b. self-fed with some difficulty = 1 point c. self-fed without any problem = 2 points	☐

SELF ASSESSMENT

17. Do they view themselves as having nutritional problems? a. major malnutrition = 0 points b. does not know or moderate malnutrition = 1 point c. no nutritional problem = 2 points	☐
18. In comparison with other people of the same age, how do they consider their health status? a. not as good = 0.0 points b. does not know = 0.5 points c. as good = 1.0 points d. better = 2.0 points	☐.☐

ASSESSMENT TOTAL (max. 30 points): ☐☐.☐

MALNUTRITION INDICATOR SCORE

≥ 24 points	well-nourished	☐
17 to 23.5 points	at risk of malnutrition	☐
< 17 points	malnourished	☐

Ref.: Guigoz Y, Vellas B and Garry PJ. 1994. Mini Nutritional Assessment: A practical assessment tool for grading the nutritional state of elderly patients. *Facts and Research in Gerontology.* Supplement #2: 15-59.

NESTLÉ NUTRITION SERVICES

Updated Version

Mini Nutritional Assessment MNA®

Last name: First name: Sex: Date:

Age: Weight, kg: Height, cm: I.D. Number:

Complete the screen by filling in the boxes with the appropriate numbers.
Add the numbers for the screen. If score is 11 or less, continue with the assessment to gain a Malnutrition Indicator Score.

Screening

A Has food intake declined over the past 3 months due to loss of appetite, digestive problems, chewing or swallowing difficulties?
0 = severe loss of appetite
1 = moderate loss of appetite
2 = no loss of appetite ☐

B Weight loss during last months
0 = weight loss greater than 3 kg (6.6 lbs)
1 = does not know
2 = weight loss between 1 and 3 kg (2.2 and 6.6 lbs)
3 = no weight loss ☐

C Mobility
0 = bed or chair bound
1 = able to get out of bed/chair but does not go out
2 = goes out ☐

D Has suffered psychological stress or acute disease in the past 3 months
0 = yes 2 = no ☐

E Neuropsychological problems
0 = severe dementia or depression
1 = mild dementia
2 = no psychological problems ☐

F Body Mass Index (BMI) (weight in kg) / (height in m)^2
0 = BMI less than 19
1 = BMI 19 to less than 21
2 = BMI 21 to less than 23
3 = BMI 23 or greater ☐

Screening score (subtotal max. 14 points) ☐ ☐

12 points or greater — Normal – not at risk – no need to complete assessment

11 points or below — Possible malnutrition – continue assessment

Assessment

G Lives independently (not in a nursing home or hospital)
0 = no 1 = yes ☐

H Takes more than 3 prescription drugs per day
0 = yes 1 = no ☐

I Pressure sores or skin ulcers
0 = yes 1 = no ☐

J How many full meals does the patient eat daily?
0 = 1 meal
1 = 2 meals
2 = 3 meals ☐

K Selected consumption markers for protein intake
- At least one serving of dairy products (milk, cheese, yogurt) per day? yes ☐ no ☐
- Two or more serving of legumes or eggs per week? yes ☐ no ☐
- Meat, fish or poultry every day yes ☐ no ☐

0.0 = if 0 or 1 yes
0.5 = if 2 yes
1.0 = if 3 yes ☐.☐

L Consumes two or more servings of fruits or vegetables per day?
0 = no 1 = yes ☐

M How much fluid (water, juice, coffee, tea, milk...) is consumed per day?
0.0 = less than 3 cups
0.5 = 3 to 5 cups
1.0 = more than 5 cups ☐.☐

N Mode of feeding
0 = unable to eat without assistance
1 = self-fed with some difficulty
2 = self-fed without any problem ☐

O Self view of nutritional status
0 = view self as being malnourished
1 = is uncertain of nutritional state
2 = views self as having no nutritional problem ☐

P In comparison with other people of the same age, how do they consider their health status?
0.0 = not as good
0.5 = does not know
1.0 = as good
2.0 = better ☐.☐

Q Mid-arm circumference (MAC) in cm
0.0 = MAC less than 21
0.5 = MAC 21 to 22
1.0 = MAC 22 or greater ☐.☐

R Calf circumference (CC) in cm
0 = CC less than 31 1 = CC 31 or greater ☐

Assessment (max. 16 points) ☐ ☐.☐

Screening score ☐ ☐

Total Assessment (max. 30 points) ☐ ☐.☐

Malnutrition Indicator Score

17 to 23.5 points — at risk of malnutrition ☐

Less than 17 points — malnourished ☐

Ref.: Guigoz Y, Vellas B and Garry PJ. 1994. Mini Nutritional Assessment: A practical assessment tool for grading the nutritional state of elderly patients. *Facts and Research in Gerontology.* Supplement #2:15-59.

Rubenstein LZ, Harker J, Guigoz Y and Vellas B. Comprehensive Geriatric Assessment (CGA) and the MNA: An Overview of CGA, Nutritional Assessment, and Development of a Shortened Version of the MNA. In: "Mini Nutritional Assessment (MNA): Research and Practice in the Elderly". Vellas B, Garry PJ and Guigoz Y, editors. Nestlé Nutrition Workshop Series. Clinical & Performance Programme, vol. 1. Karger, Bâle, in press.

08.98 USA

Mini Nutritional Assessment (MNA): Research and Practice in the Elderly:
B. Vellas; P.J. Garry; Y. Guigoz (eds),
Nestlé Nutrition Workshop Series Clinical & Performance Programme, Vol. 1, pp. 159–176,
Nestec Ltd.; Vevey/S. Karger AG, Basel, © 1999.

Posters

Mini Nutritional Assessment in Nursing Home Residents

M. Molaschi, M. Massaia, A. Pallavicino di Ceva, F. Nicoletti, E. Ferrario, M. Ponzetto and G. Cappa

Department of Medical and Surgical Disciplines, Geriatric Section, University of Turin, Turin, Italy

Our aim in this study was to evaluate the MNA in a population of institutionalized elderly people, and its correlation with functional and nutritional variables.

The study group included 100 subjects, 24 men and 76 women, with mean age 85.4 ± 9.2 (SD) years; their mean period of stay in a nursing home was 5.3 years. The score of the sample in the short portable mental status questionnaire (SPMSQ) was 6.7 ± 2.9, and in the activities of daily living (ADL) scale the lost functions were 4.7 ± 1.5.

Serum albumin, transferrin, total cholesterol, triglycerides, hemoglobin, and lymphocyte count were evaluated. Linear correlation coefficient analysis (SPSS/PC) was performed.

The malnutrition indicator score identified 19 well-nourished subjects while 60 were at risk of malnutrition and 21 were malnourished. The total assessment score was positively correlated with serum albumin ($r = +0.392$; $p < 0.001$), transferrin ($r = +0.346$: $p < 0.001$), and hemoglobin ($r = +0.270$; $p < 0.01$). A negative correlation was found with age ($r = -0.271$; $p < 0.01$), mental impairment based on the SPMSQ score ($r = -0.589$; $p < 0.001$), and loss of autonomy expressed by the number of lost functions in the ADL ($r = -0.602$; $p < 0.001$).

With regard to each item of the MNA, body mass index was negatively correlated with the SPMSQ score ($r = -0.272$; $p < 0.01$) and the number of dependent ADL functions ($r = -0.273$; $p < 0.01$). Calf circumference was negatively correlated with age ($r = -0.350$; $p < 0.001$), the SPMSQ score ($r = -0.369$; $p < 0.001$), and the number of dependent ADL functions ($r = -0.261$; $p < 0.01$). The absence of psychological stress or acute disease in the past 3 months was positively related to serum albumin ($r = +0.257$; $p < 0.01$) and transferrin ($r = +0.239$; $p < 0.01$). Mobility was positively correlated with serum albumin ($r = +0.293$; $p < 0.01$) and negatively with the number of dependent ADL functions ($r = -0.561$; $p < 0.001$). Protein intake was negatively related to the number of dependent ADL functions ($r = -0.254$; $p < 0.01$); the mode of feeding showed a negative correlation with the SPMSQ score

($r = -0.487$; $p < 0.001$) and the loss of autonomy in the ADL ($r = -0.548$; $p < 0.001$), while it positively influenced serum albumin ($r = +0.368$; $p < 0.001$) and hemoglobin ($r = +0.254$; $p < 0.01$). Finally, age ($r = -0.240$; $p < 0.01$) and mental impairment ($r = -0.429$; $p < 0.001$) were significantly related to the daily intake of fluids.

Our study shows that there are significant correlations between MNA items and functional and nutritional variables. MNA is a useful tool for evaluating nutritional status in elderly people living in nursing homes.

Malnutrition in Elderly Care – An Expression of Aging and Disease or of Insufficient Nutritional Routines?

Anja Saletti, Lennarth Johansson, Elinor Yifer-Lindgren, Gun-Britt Håkansson, Agneta Kling and Tommy Cederholm

Swedish National Board of Health and Welfare, Stockholm, Sweden

Aims – Almost 100,000 people in Sweden, who require various degrees of help, live in "special housing forms" run by local municipalities, that is, service flats (SF), sheltered homes (SH), old people's homes (OPH), and nursing homes (NH). In this investigation we used the MNA technique to assess the nutritional status of a representative sample of this population, who are often elderly and have chronic diseases.

Methods – The study population consisted of all individuals in special housing in the municipalities of Falkenberg (n = 551), Robertsfors (n = 198), and Katarina-Sofia in Stockholm (n = 286). In the three study areas, 8%, 16%, and 18%, respectively, dropped out. The average age of the 872 individuals examined was 84.5 ± 8 years; 69% were women, and 349 (40%), 96 (11%), 261 (30%), and 166 (19%) of the individuals lived in SF, SH, OPH, and NH, respectively. Nutritional status was assessed using the MNA scale, consisting of 18 point-weighted questions divided into four categories. These include anthropomorphic measurements (for example, body mass index (BMI, kg/m^2, normal range 20–25)), "global assessment," dietary assessment (for example, menus, appetite), and the individual's subjective assessment. The maximum number of points is 30; <17 is viewed as "malnutrition" and 17–23.5 as "risk for malnutrition."

Results – MNA <17, that is, "malnutrition," was noted in 36% of the study population. Divided by housing type, the MNA score was <17 in 21% (SF), 38% (SH), 33% (OPH), and 71% (NH). The corresponding percentages for MNA score of 17–23.5 ("risk for malnutrition") were 49%, 51%, 57%, and 29%, respectively. For MNA scores of ≥24, the percentages were 30%, 10%, 10%, and 0%, respectively. Average BMI values were 24.2 ± 5 (SF), 23.9 ± 4 (SH), 22.6 ± 5 (OPH), and 22.3 ± 4 (NH). BMI values ≤20 were found in 18% (SF), 19% (SH), 25% (OPH), and 33% (NH), respectively ($p < 0.001$). The coefficient of correlation between MNA and BMI was $r = 0.5$, $p < 0.001$. The age of the individuals in the four housing types was 84 ± 9 (SF), 83 ± 7 (SH), 86 ± 7 (OPH), and 84 ± 8 years (NH), $p < 0.05$. The correlations between age and MNA and between age and BMI were significant but low, $r = 0.1$ ($p < 0.01$) and $r = 0.14$ ($p < 0.001$), respectively.

Conclusions – According to the MNA, the occurrence of malnutrition appears to be high within elderly care as run by local municipalities. The highest prevalence is in NH (70%) and the lowest in SF (20%). Age and disease mean that malnutrition is probably unavoidable to a certain extent. The results point to the need for reappraisal of the nutritional routines within elderly care but further studies are necessary to assess the degree to which the nutritional disturbances shown are reversible.

Mini Nutritional Assessment in Elderly People Living at Home in Warsaw

Jadwiga Charzewska, Elzbieta Chabros, Malgorzata Rogalska-Niedzwiedz, Bozena Wajszczyk, Maria Wartanowicz and Swiatoslaw Ziemlanski

National Food and Nutrition Institute, Warsaw, Poland

Aim – The purpose of this study was to assess the predicting capacity of the MNA instrument for the rapid evaluation of malnutrition in the present economic and social situation in Poland. The study was carried out in 1997 among a random selection of 43 males and 59 females aged 75 years, living freely at home in Warsaw.

Methods – The following were assessed: MNA score, energy and nutrient intakes by the 24-hour recall method, health status, anthropometry, and biomedical analyses (for example, hemoglobin, vitamin C).

Results – Average body mass index (BMI) was 27.6 kg/m^2 in males and 28.5 kg/m^2 in females; energy intake was 2,065 kcal in males and 1,494 kcal in females; protein intake was 0.9 g/kg and 0.8 g/kg; fat intake was 83 g and 58 g (cholesterol 290 mg and 253 mg), respectively. Intakes below the recommended daily allowances (RDA) were found for Ca, Mg, Fe, vitamin B2, vitamin B6, and free folacin. MNA scores were: malnourished, 0% males and 2% females; at risk of malnutrition, 14% males and 17% females; well-nourished, 86% males and 81% females. The frequency of health disorders, anemia, deficient levels vitamin C, and low intakes of energy and nutrients were analyzed in these three groups.

Conclusions – This study confirms the value of the MNA in free-living elderly Polish people. However, there is a need to undertake further validation of score indicators, especially high BMI, for the subjective assessment of self perceived health, and also to discuss thresholds.

Evaluating the NSI (Nutrition Screening Initiative Checklist) and MNA as Tools for Assessing the Nutritional Situation of Elderly People

C.P.G.M. de Groot, A. van Lier, J. Prompers and W.A. van Staveren
for the SENECA investigators

Two short questionnaires aiming at a rapid assessment of the nutritional status of elderly people have been tested by comparing cumulative scores with data on dietary intake, anthropometric measurements, blood biochemistry, lifestyle, and physical and mental performance. The questionnaires of interest are the nutrition screening initiative checklist (NSI) from the United States and the MNA as developed in France. Information similar to the questions of the NSI and MNA lists was collected by the Survey in Europe on Nutrition and the Elderly, a Concerted Action (SENECA). This study included 1,161 elderly men and women born between and 1913 and 1918, mostly living at home, whose diet, lifestyle, and health have been studied twice: in 1989 and in 1993. The MNA classified 55% of the examinees as well-nourished, 44% as at risk of malnutrition, and 1% as undernourished. The NSI categorized the elderly people differently: 11% as well-nourished, 42% as at moderate nutritional risk, 48% as at high nutritional risk. Incidental differences emerged for biochemical indices (serum albumin, hemoglobin, lymphocyte count, serum lipids, serum vitamins), intakes of energy and protein, and anthropometric characteristics between MNA categories and between NSI categories. Using serum albumin values (<30 g/l) and lymphocyte counts (<1,500/ml^3) as standards, the specificity and sensitivity of both instruments for identifying at-risk groups were below 0.6. Only with body weight loss (≥ 10%) as a criterion were higher sensitivities (0.96 (MNA), 0.75 (NSI)) and specificities found (0.60 (MNA), 0.54 (NSI)). It is concluded that the usefulness of both assessment tools for a healthy elderly population needs further evaluation.

Monitoring Malnutrition in Home Nursing: A Three-Step Model Using ADL and MNA

D. Ridder, H. Vandenbroele, R. Wouters and L. Geys

White and Yellow Cross of Belgium, Brussels, Belgium

Aims – The White and Yellow Cross of Belgium carried out a study on patients receiving home nursing, the so-called Nutritional Assessment and Monitoring of Elderly study (NAME study) [Wouters, Vandenbroele, *et al.*, 1997]. The aim of this study was to determine whether a three-step monitoring model in home nursing is feasible: (1) case finding using the activities of daily life scale (ADL) [Katz, 1961]; (2) screening using the MNA [Guigoz *et al.*, 1994], and (3) applying a nursing protocol for malnutrition. This paper deals with the validity study of steps one and two.

Methods – In a random cluster sample of elderly patients over 60 years of age, interviews were carried out in November 1995 by trained nurses. This survey included sociodemographic data, nursing data, ADL, instrumental ADL, and dietary intake. Research questions were aimed at: (1) the prevalence of malnutrition according to the MNA; (2) the dietary intake of the home nursing patients according to a memory-friendly food frequency questionnaire [De Ridder, 1997] as a concurrent validation of the MNA, and (3) validating case finding on the basis of ADL, using the MNA as the criterion. For the statistical analysis we used SAS software, and food consumption was converted into energy and nutrients using the Dutch food tables.

Results – General Findings: 529 patients (69% women); age 77.7 ± 8.8 years, BMI 25.7 ± 4.8 kg/m^2. The mean energy intake was 1,722 ± 571 kcal. On average, 35% did not reach a daily intake of 1,500 kcal. Separate results of the intake of protein, vitamin B1, vitamin B2, vitamin B6, vitamin C, Fe, Ca, Zn, food fiber, and liquid are available. We observed a high mean protein intake of 75 ± 28 g/day. Insufficient intakes were observed for vitamins, minerals, and fluids (a daily average of 1 liter of fluid less than recommended). According to the MNA screening, 6.2% of the patients have malnutrition (MNA < 17), 45.5% are at risk of malnutrition (MNA 17–23.5), and 48.3% are well-nourished (MNA ≥ 24).

Specific Research Findings: We showed that case finding for the MNA can easily be done using an ADL score of ≥ 15 as an indicator for MNA, with a sensitivity of 79% and a specificity of 82%. If this ADL score criterion is used, we found that MNA was indicated in 32% of our patients. If we used the MNA in this group without selection by ADL score, we found a maximum of 6.2% undernutrition; in the group with an ADL score of ≥ 15 we found 15% malnutrition. In the same way, without a preliminary ADL score we found that 48.3% were well-nourished; in the group with an ADL score ≥ 15, we found only 27% were well-nourished.

Conclusions – For systematic screening with the MNA, the scope of the screening can be reduced to one third of all elderly patients in Belgian home care by selecting only individuals with an ADL score ≥ 15. Future research should validate the use of a nursing protocol for malnutrition in the proposed three-step framework.

Nutritional Assessment in Primary Care – A Pilot Study

Hedi Decrey, Fabienne Vauthier, Luc Tappy and Christophe Büla

Policlinique Medicale Universitaire, Lausanne, Switzerland

Nutritional intervention should occur early in the course of undernutrition to be effective. In elderly outpatients, however, nutritional screening is rarely carried out routinely. Strategies are therefore needed to increase the physician's awareness of this assessment. The objectives of this pilot study were: (1) to determine the nutritional status of a population of community-dwelling elderly people visiting a university teaching hospital medical outpatient clinic, and (2) to test the feasibility of the use of the MNA in an outpatient setting. All patients aged 65 years or older scheduled for an appointment at the clinic during a period of 1 week were offered the opportunity to have a MNA. The assessment was conducted by a nurse specialized in nutrition. Fifty-three of 67 eligible patients participated in the study, 33 women and 20 men. Mean age was 79.9 ± 6.8 years. One man was malnourished according to the MNA score (MNA <17) and 22.6% (four men and eight women) were at risk of malnutrition (MNA 17–23.5). The proportion of subjects malnourished or at risk increased with age from 9.1% to 32% and 50% in the 65–74, 75–84, and 85+ year age groups, respectively. In addition, in only one of these patients did the medical file specially mention the patient's nutritional status. We conclude that risk of malnutrition is common in this elderly population visiting a primary care facility, but the problem is rarely identified. Strategies to increase recognition of this condition in primary care settings are therefore needed.

Copper, Zinc, and Magnesium Blood Levels in Healthy People: Comparison between Elderly People and Younger People

L. Del Corso[a], D. Moruzzo[a], F. Pentimone[a], A.M. Romanelli[c], M.A. Protti[c], V. Pagni[a], F. Pastine[a] and L. Ruocco[b]

Istituto Clinica Medica II, U.O. di [a]Geriatria e di [b]Laboratorio, University of Pisa, Italy; [c]Istituto di Fisiologia Clinica, Reparto Epidemiologia e Biostatistica, C.N.R. Pisa, Italy

Nutrition plays a central role in the maintenance of health in elderly people, who are sometimes at risk of inadequate nutrient intake. The aim of this study was to clarify the influence of age on blood levels of copper (Cu), zinc (Zn), and intracellular and extracellular magnesium (iMg; eMg).

Inclusion criteria – Healthy subjects, males (M) and females (F), of any age. Cu values (70–140 µg/dl for M, 85–155 µg/dl for F), Zn (55–120 µg/dl), and iMg (1.97–2.96 mmol/l) were measured by atomic absorption spectrophotometry, eMg (0.74–1.23 mmol/l) by a colorimetric method, and the ceruloplasmin (0.99–3.96 µmol/l) by nephelometry.

Statistical analysis – Data are expressed as mean ± SD, and were analyzed by Student's *t* test for unpaired data, χ^2 test, and simple linear regression.

Results – 143 subjects (20–102 years) were enrolled in two groups, above and below 65 years: 107 younger subjects (67 M, 43.8 ± 11.7 years, and 40 F, 40.2 ± 10.1 years); 36 elderly subjects (22 M, 70.5 ± 5.5 years, and 14 F, 87.7 ± 10.5 years), with a homogeneous sex distribution (χ^2 0.97; NS). Micronutrient levels in the elderly and the younger subjects, respectively, were: Cu 117.5 ± 17.0 and 102.5 ± 19.6 µg/dl ($p < 0.001$); Zn 113.3 ± 14.9 and 118.0 ± 17.3 µg/dl (NS); iMg 2.12 ± 0.20 and 2.07 ± 0.20 mmol/l (NS); eMg 0.89 ± 0.10 and 0.84 ± 0.10 mmol/l ($p < 0.05$). We found abnormal levels of Cu in 5%, of Zn in 36%, of iMg in 23.3%, homogeneously distributed in the two groups (NS; χ^2 0.08, 0.17, and

0.04, respectively). All subjects with abnormally low Cu were in the younger group. Abnormal levels of eMg were found in 18%, mostly low values (89.5%), especially in younger subjects (χ^2 4.06; $p < 0.05$). In the two groups, RBC, Hb, iron, transferrin, and ferritin were homogeneously distributed by gender; total proteins and albumin were higher in the younger subjects ($p < 0.05$ and $p < 0.01$, respectively). Body mass index values in the older and in the younger subjects, respectively, were: (M) 24.0 ± 2.8 and 24.2 ± 2.7 kg/m^2 (NS), (F) 29.4 ± 8.3 and 21.3 ± 2.9 kg/m^2 ($p < 0.01$). No correlation was found between any micronutrient and age. Splitting by gender in the total population, Cu levels were higher in the elderly and ceruloplasmin higher only in old males; in the younger group, Cu levels were homogeneous and ceruloplasmin was higher in females; in the older group Cu levels were higher in females and ceruloplasmin in males. Although the elderly group seemed at risk for low intakes of micronutrients, we found no deficit of micronutrients and nutritional indices were normal in all subjects.

Published data are contradictory, probably because it is difficult to find really healthy elderly people and to prove micronutrient deficiency using current laboratory tests. The already described age-related increase in Cu may cause faster atherosclerosis and fibrosis of small vessels, linked to enhanced lipid peroxidation. The contradictory data on the Cu/ceruloplasmin/gender relation cannot be explained by a hormone influence, but suggest that blood Cu and ceruloplasmin may not be markers of Cu status. The higher levels of eMg in the elderly group strengthens the possibility that the commonly found Mg deficiency is linked to drugs interfering with nutrient absorption and utilization and not to the aging process itself. Both the older and the younger subjects had Zn levels similar to those found in previous studies. These results suggest that healthy elderly people usually have a balanced diet; acute and chronic diseases and/or function impairment may cause undernutrition or malnutrition.

MNA in a Population of Frail Elderly People

L.M. Donini, M.R. De Felice, F. Deon, C. Moretti and L. De Bernardini

Istituto Geriatrico "Villa delle Querce", Nemi, Italy

The predictive value of the MNA was evaluated in a population of frail elderly people admitted to long-term hospital care, in comparison with a nutritional global assessment (NGA). NGA is used as standard and is inserted into the comprehensive geriatric assessment that we carry out in all our patients on admission; it includes both anthropometric measurements (triceps skinfold, cutoff 10 mm for men, 13.2 mm for women, and muscle circumference, cutoff 20.2 cm for men, 18.6 cm for women) and biochemical indices (albumin, cutoff 30 g/l, transferrin, cutoff 2 g/l, and lymphocyte count, cutoff 1,500/mm^3) [Donini LM, *et al: Age Nutr* 1994; 3: 182].

All patients admitted consecutively to our institute from January to July 1997 were entered into the study. There were 45 men aged 76.8 ± 12 years and 54 women aged 80.8 ± 9 years. All had multiple organ disease (3.8 ± 1) and for this reason were taking 4.7 ± 2 drugs daily; most (72%) were functionally impaired and 55% were moderately or severely demented.

The prevalence of malnutrition by NGA evaluation was 78.8%. Twenty subjects were classified as "at risk of malnutrition" by MNA; of the remaining 79 subjects, 13 (16.5%) were misclassified by MNA. The sensitivity and positive predictive value of MNA were 98.5% and 84.4%, respectively.

We had 12 (15.2%) false-positive MNA assessments: for these subjects MNA scores, especially in the "general" and "self-assessment" sections, were very low and not different from the scores for malnourished patients in the same sections. We believe that functional and cognitive impairment can affect the scores of these sections. On the other hand, as was observed in our sample, these impairments are not necessarily correlated with malnutrition, at least in their early stage. In spite of this, MNA is a valid tool for evaluating elderly people at risk of malnutrition because of its high sensitivity and ease of administration (since it does not require a specialized nutritional assessment team).

Study of Determinants of the Response to Influenza Vaccine in Institutionalized Elderly People

T. Fülöp[a], J.R. Wagner[b], A. Khalil[a], J. Weber[c], L. Trottier[a] and H. Payette[a]

[a] *Research Center in Gerontology and Geriatrics,* [b] *Department of Nuclear Medicine and Radiobiology, University Institute of Geriatrics, Sherbrooke;* [c] *Surveillance, Influenza and Viral Exanthemata, LCDC Virus Laboratory, Ottawa, Canada*

Influenza is a major health problem among elderly subjects in industrialized countries, mainly among nursing home residents. The aim of this study was to evaluate some aspects of the nutritional status of institutionalized elderly people in relation to the response to influenza vaccination. Certain aspects of the cellular immune response were also investigated. Twenty-three patients participated in the study. All the patients were vaccinated on day 0. The vaccination was done with Fluviral®, 1994–95 preparation: A/Shangdong/09/93, A/Texas/36/91, B/Panama/45/90. We assessed prevaccination antibody titer, nutritional status by MNA and by biochemical indices, and lymphocyte proliferation at the same time. On day 28, the postvaccination antibody titer was determined. Determination of antibody titers against the various influenza antigens in the pre- and postvaccination period was carried out by hemagglutination. Eleven elderly people were responsive (a fourfold increase in any of the virus antigens), while 12 were not. We have shown that hemoglobin, hematocrit, total protein, iron and vitamin E levels, DHEA level, and the cellular immune response were significantly decreased in the nonresponsive group. These variables might play a role in the influenza vaccine responsiveness of the elderly. These results may help in the design of intervention studies for improving the immune response by achieving optimal nutritional status, mainly in frail elderly people.

Diagnostic and Prognostic Efficiency of the MNA Nutritional Scale in Geriatric Medicine

C. Gazzotti, A. Pepinster, J. Petermans and A. Albert

Blv. du XII de Ligne, Department of Gerontology, CHR Citadelle, Liège, Belgium

Aims – (1) to estimate the prevalence of undernutrition in a geriatric population hospitalized with an acute illness; (2) to study the correlation between the MNA score and the autonomy score measured by the Katz scale; (3) to establish the reliability of the MNA score in predicting admission to nursing homes after discharge from hospital; and (4) to compare the MNA score between groups, survivors and nonsurvivors.

Methods – MNA was determined in 175 hospital inpatients (113 women and 62 men) aged 79.7 ± 8.45 years. The Katz score on admission and at discharge, the number of different medications, and clinical course of the patients were recorded by two geriatricians.

Results – The mean MNA score was 20.5 ± 5.1. There was no significant correlation between MNA score and age, sex, or height, but there was a correlation between MNA score and weight ($r = 0.45$; $p < 0.01$) and body mass index (BMI; $r = 0.44$; $p < 0.0001$). A significant inverse relation was found between MNA and Katz score on admission ($r = -0.37$; $p < 0.0001$) and on discharge ($r = -0.52$; $p < 0.0001$). The mean number of drugs taken was 5.17 ± 2.82 and this number was negatively correlated with the MNA score ($r = -0.23$; $p < 0.05$); poor values on the MNA score were related to steroids, laxatives, and sedative drugs. The MNA score was significantly lower in elderly people who came from a nursing home than in those who lived at home: 18.4 ± 5.1 *vs.* 22.3 ± 4.7 ($p < 0.001$). During hospitalization, 6.3% died. There was a significant difference between the survivors and nonsurvivors in terms of age ($p = 0.045$) and weight ($p = 0.022$). The MNA value for the group which died was significantly lower (14.1) than for the group which survived (20.9). Finally, our study showed that the MNA score was not a good predictor of disposal on discharge from hospital.

Conclusions – The MNA assessment is a reliable tool. Our study showed an inverse correlation between MNA and Katz score, as well as between MNA score and the number of different drugs taken (steroids, laxatives, and sedatives). The MNA scores were better in subjects living at home than in those living in nursing home. There was a significant correlation between MNA score and the risk of death during hospital admission. The MNA can hardly be used as a hint for future placement.

Malnutrition Risk Screening by the MNA for Elderly Patients in a Rehabilitation Ward after Femoral Neck Fracture

M.A. Blanchon, O. Beauchet, M. Roy, M.F. Odelin and R. Gonthier

Service de Gérontologie, Clinique Hôpital de la Charité, Saint-Etienne, France

Aims – Postoperative care in elderly populations with femoral fractures requires re-education and rehabilitation, but malnutrition needs to be detected because of its effects in retarding healing and reducing muscular strength.

Methods – In a prospective study, we estimated nutritional risk by MNA in 15 elderly patients (mean age 86.8 ± 4.7 years) hospitalized in a rehabilitation ward after surgery for femoral neck fractures, and compared them with a control group of 15 patients in the same age range (mean age 81.9 ± 5.7 years) in a day-stay hospital for minor procedures.

Results – The operated patients were more likely to be malnourished than the day-case patients. Operated patients had a mean body mass index of 19.9 ± 3.5 *vs.* 24.3 ± 4.6 in the controls ($p = 0.006$). Weight in the fracture group was 50.6 ± 9.3 kg *vs.* 60.3 ± 12.2 kg in the controls ($p = 0.02$). The mean MNA of the fracture group was 15 ± 4.8, that is, in the frank malnutrition range, compared with 24.3 ± 4.5 in the control group ($p = 0.001$) – nearly in the well-nourished range (MNA >24). There was a greater difference in calf circumference (fracture group 26.5 ± 2.8 cm *vs.* controls 32.9 ± 4.8 cm; $p = 0.0001$) than in arm circumference (21.9 ± 2.4 cm *vs.* 24.7 ± 4 cm; $p = 0.03$).

Conclusions – The MNA is a practical tool for nutrition screening. It is possible to identify undernutrition in surgical patients. This assessment is essential to identify the need for protein supplementation and to optimize functional capacity.

Validation of a Spanish Version of the MNA in a Mexican Population

M. Flores Castro, L. Gutierrez-Robledo, K. Romero and C. Llaca

Instituto Nacional de la Nutrición "Salvador Zubirán", Tlalpan, Mexico

Aim – Nutritional disorders are common in the elderly. About 60% of individuals in our clinic show evidence of a nutritional disorder, but since anthropometric, biochemical and dietary assessments are expensive and time consuming, and since physicians usually do not have the skills needed to perform a satisfactory nutritional assessment in their patients, there is a need for simple screening instruments in Spanish for this purpose.

Methods – The study was a diagnostic test evaluation in a geriatric population from a geriatric consultation clinic (60 years of age and over). Sample size, calculated from a diagnostic test evaluation formula, was 219. These patients underwent a global nutritional assessment (GNA), including anthropometric assessment, dietary assessment, serum albumin, cholesterol, lymphocyte count and hemoglobin level, together with "blind" scoring of the MNA.

Results – 65 men and 164 women were assessed; mean age of the sample was 79 years, and 51% were between 75 and 85 years. On GNA evaluation we found that 23% of our population fulfilled diagnostic criteria for malnutrition and 77% were normal or overweight. When correlating the results of the GNA with the MNA we found that all cases who were malnourished on GNA scored <23.5 points on MNA. Of these, 47% had a score of <17 and 53% between 17 and 23.5. In contrast, 77% of subjects classified as being normal or overweight had MNA scores of between 17 and 23.5, putting them in the risk category according to the originally proposed scoring system. Only 9% identified as "normal" had scores <17 which misclassified them as malnourished.

Conclusions – The MNA seems a useful instrument for screening of undernutrition. When performing an ROC analysis the best cutoff point for our results was 19. With this cutoff point we had a sensitivity of 89% and a specificity of 60%. It must be stressed that 77% of our normals had low scores which would classify them as at risk. We are conducting a follow-up of these patients to identify whether there is a deterioration in their nutritional status, since the low MNA score could mean that there are risk factors present that could eventually lead to malnutrition. It must nevertheless be emphasized that 100% of patients with malnutrition had scores of <23.5, showing very good discrimination, and also that the MNA is a fast and cheap instrument.

Nutritional Status, Pathology, and Outcome in a Geriatric Hospital Inpatient Population

E. Joosten, B. Vanderelst, S. Christiaens and N. Peeters

Division of Geriatric Medicine, University Hospitals, K.U. Leuven, Belgium

The nutritional status of 155 consecutive geriatric patients (mean age 83 years, 51 males and 104 females) was assessed on admission by means of MNA, dietary intake, anthropometric methods (body mass index, BMI; triceps skinfold, TSF; mid-upper arm circumference, MAC) and laboratory (serum albumin) measurements. The aim of the study was to correlate the MNA with: (1) the principal clinical diagnosis on admission; (2) a long stay (≥30 days) in hospital, and (3) in-hospital survival. According to the MNA, 40 patients (26%) were undernourished on admission (score <17), 81 (52%) were at risk (score between

17 and 23.5), and 34 (22%) were well-nourished (score >23.5). The table shows the distribution of albumin, BMI, MAC, and TSF (<10th percentile of a healthy elderly control group), and mean energy intake, according to nutritional status.

	MNA score		
	<17	≥17 to 23.5	≥24
Albumin <3.5	23/40	28/81	14/34
BMI <20 kg/m^2	17/40	9/81	1/34
MAC <P 10	34/40	47/81	13/34
TSF <P10	21/40	18/81	4/34
Mean energy intake (SD), kcal/day	1,753 (496)	1,970 (458)	2,305 (490)

Of the 155 patients, 32 had a cardiovascular disorder, 29 an acute infection, 18 a malignant tumor, 11 dementia/depression, and 65 another disorder. The mean (SD) MNA score in these subgroups was 20.6 (4.5), 18.4 (6.2), 16.8 (4.3), 17.9 (5.4), and 20.4 (4.5), respectively (NS). The mean MNA score in the 12 patients who died during hospitalization (17.7) was comparable with the MNA score in the survivors (19.6; $p = 0.18$), and seven patients in the former group had an MNA score of >17. The MNA score of the patients with a hospital stay of ≥30 days (19.6) was also comparable with that of the patients with a stay of <30 days (19.2), and the proportion of patients who were malnourished, at risk, and well-nourished was comparable in the two subgroups. There were 17 patients with iron deficiency anemia, 29 with anemia of chronic disease, 14 with another cause of anemia, and 95 were not anemic. The mean MNA scores and the proportions of patients in the three MNA categories were comparable between these four groups.

Conclusions – Using the MNA test, the prevalence of patients who are undernourished or at risk of malnutrition is substantial in a geriatric hospital inpatient population. However, the MNA score was comparable between the main disease categories, and nutritional status did not seem to influence survival and length of hospital stay.

Role of Immune Status in MNA in the Elderly

V.K. Khavinson and D.V. Solovieva

Institute of Bioregulation and Gerontology, St. Petersburg, Russia

The purpose of this study was to investigate immune indices in geriatric patients of various nutritional status. One hundred and twenty patients (30 males and 90 females) aged 60–85 years were divided into two groups according to MNA score. The patients in the first group were malnourished (score <17), and the second group was well-nourished (score ≥24).

All patients had investigations of immune indices (CD3, CD4, CD8, CD4/CD8, CD20, Con A-induced leukocyte migration inhibition test, PHA-induced PBMC proliferation test, phagocytic reactions).

The results showed a decrease in lymphokine production in the malnourished patients (Con A-induced leukocyte migration inhibition reduced by 27% and PHA-induced PBMC proliferation by 34%; CD4/CD8 index decreased by 38% comparing with a standard).

Thus there are diagnostic immunological signs in elderly people identified as malnourished by the MNA.

MNA in Residential Home Residents

L. Hrabinská, Š. Krajcík, A. Sobolová and M. Šauša

Geriatric Department of the Postgraduate Medical School, Bratislava, Slovakia

One hundred elderly people (20 men and 80 women) over 65 years living in a residential home were assessed by the MNA.

41% were at risk of malnutrition and 5% were malnourished. Malnutrition was more frequent in men (65% *vs.* 35%). More than three drugs were used by 75.6% persons at risk of malnutrition, by 60% of malnourished individuals, and by 40.7% of those not at risk. Low meat consumption was found in 65.8% of people at risk of malnutrition, in 75% of malnourished individuals, and in 53.7% of well-nourished individuals. Low milk consumption was found in 51% of persons at risk, in 60% of malnourished people, and in 24.1% of people not at risk. A low intake of fruit and vegetables was found in 43.9% of persons at risk, in 20% of malnourished people, and in 29.6% of well-nourished people. A low intake of fluids was found in all the malnourished people, in 90% of the people at risk, and in none of the well-nourished people. A low body mass index was found in 75% of malnourished people, in 36.5% people at risk, and in 3.7% of people not at risk. Decreased appetite was found in 75% of malnourished people, in 19.5% of those at risk, and in 7.4% of those not at risk. Poor health status self-assessment was found in 20% of malnourished people, in 51.2% of those at risk, and in 11.1% of those not at risk.

Health and Nutritional Status of Retirement Home Residents

M. Adamska-Skula and R. Lutynski

Department of Hygiene and Ecology, Collegium Medicum, Jagiellonian University, Kraków, Poland

The aim of the study was to define the state of health and nutritional status in residents of retirement homes. One hundred and seven subjects, aged 65–104 years, living in selected welfare facilities in the Kraków region, were asked about their health complaints, medical history, mobility and daily activity, dietary patterns, and their self-assessment of their health. They were also examined and had anthropometry.

The most common health disorders were atherosclerotic hypertension, coronary heart disease, congestive heart failure, peripheral vascular disease, and arthroses. Mobility was at a satisfactory level but there was a low level of physical and daily living activity.

Body mass index (BMI) values often exceeded recommended levels: BMI >25 (below 30) was found in 27% of the subjects, and BMI >30 in 25%. Other anthropometric measures (triceps skinfold, midarm circumference) did not confirm such a high prevalence of obesity. On the basis of the MNA, most of people examined were at risk of malnutrition (62%) or malnourished (21%); only 17% were assessed as well-nourished.

In conclusion, health disorders diagnosed in this group were typical diseases of the elderly. Nutritional status was poor, and the low level of activity calls for action to increase the physical and mental engagement of these retirement home residents.

With respect to methodology, the BMI seemed insufficient as an index of nutritional status in the elderly, mainly owing to posture changes; substitution of knee height or arm length might be required. It would also be useful to widen the MNA scale, with higher values reflecting cases of energy overnutrition.

Nutritional Status in the Jerusalem 70-Year-Olds Longitudinal Study: Relation to Cognitive Function, Mobility, Morbidity, and Mortality

Y. Maaravi, E. Berry, A. Cohen, G. Ginsberg and J. Stessman

Department of Rehabilitation and Geriatrics, Hadassah University Hospital, Mt. Scopus Campus, Jerusalem, Israel

The first stage of the Jerusalem Longitudinal Cohort Study gathered extensive demographic, social and health data on a large representative sample of the city's 70-year-olds, including nutritional variables. Medical examination, anthropometric profile, functional testing, cognitive status, and laboratory investigations were included. Morbidity was assessed, including hospital admission and emergency room attendance rates. This information was used to establish a numerical nutritional assessment (NA) score, a modified form of the MNA, the reliability of which has already been validated.

Based on an NA score of >24, 91% of the study population were in good nutritional state, 8.3% were at risk of malnutrition, and 0.7% were malnourished. There was a significant positive relation between NA score and ADL, as well as cognitive status, and a strong relation between NA score and visits to the family physician, visits to the emergency room in the preceding year, and hospital admissions in the 2 years after the study. A reverse relation, although not statistically significant, was found between NA score and the 2-year post-study mortality.

We propose that the nutritional state is a major determinant of quality of life in the elderly and therefore should be part of any geriatric assessment. Population surveys of elderly people are needed to identify and treat those at risk.

Decreased Activities of Daily Living Are Associated with Measures of Undernutrition in Community-Living Elderly Subjects

N. McDowell [a], A. Murphy [b] and I.M. Rea [b]

[a] *School of Public Policy, Economics and Law, University of Ulster;*
[b] *Department of Geriatric Medicine, Queen's University of Belfast, Northern Ireland*

In community-living elderly people >85 years of age, we have previously identified evidence of malnutrition using the MNA. In this pilot study we investigated whether socioeconomic factors had any role in nutritional compromise.

Nutritional status was assessed using the MNA method in a group of 17 elderly subjects living at home (four males, 13 females, mean age 85 years) and 13 students (seven males, six females, mean age 21 years). Subjects were categorized as well-nourished, at risk, or malnourished. All subjects completed a simple questionnaire about living alone, mobility indicators, food preparation and eating, teeth, swallowing, food expenditure, milk delivery, smoking, alcohol, and previous health. The MNA showed two elderly subjects to be malnourished, three to be at risk of malnutrition, while one student was malnourished and another was at risk. Categorical variables were compared between elderly and young groups and showed elderly people more likely to live alone ($p = 0.0007$), to have reduced mobility ($p = 0.06$), to have no teeth ($p < 0.0001$), and to drink less alcohol ($p = 0.0006$) than the students, but to show no significant differences in food expenditure ($p = 0.65$), delivery of milk to the home ($p = 0.08$), or smoking ($p = 0.55$). MNA categories of nutritional assessment were entered into a logistic regression model together with categorical variables. The most important factors influencing nutrition category were the food preparation index and mobility factors, or both.

Nutritional compromise occurs in apparently well elderly people who live in the community and is related to their functional status rather than to economic factors.

Prevalence of Malnutrition in HIV-Positive Outpatients: Evaluation of the MNA

M.A. Piquet[a], E. Stoppard[a], V. Niklas[b], M. Alberti[b], S. Laffely[b], J. Von Overbeck[b], F. Donzallaz[a] and M. Roulet[a]

[a] *Unit of Clinical Nutrition,* [b] *AIDS Outpatients Clinic, University Hospital, Lausanne, Switzerland*

Aim – To examine the prevalence of malnutrition in an AIDS outpatient population with a view to finding a reasonably accurate, noninvasive method of assessing malnutrition in these patients for use in the clinical setting.

Methods – A nutritional assessment was made in 100 consecutive HIV-positive patients using body mass index (BMI), mid-arm muscle circumference, bioelectric impedance analysis, and two questionnaires: the MNA and the nutrition risk score (NRS).

Results – 19% of the patients were malnourished, 20% were at risk of malnutrition, and 61% were well-nourished. Nutritional status was not related to age, sex, ways of HIV transmission, or number of years since diagnosis. Nutritional status was positively correlated with AIDS stages, assessed by CDC staging. All but one of the malnourished and at-risk patients had a CD4 count of $<500/mm^3$. Using bioelectric impedance analysis as a reference, the sensitivities of MNA and NRS were 67% and 41%, respectively. BMI and mid-arm muscle circumference showed excellent correlation with dry lean body mass assessed by bioelectric impedance analysis ($r = 0.72$ and $r = 0.75$, respectively), while the correlation with MNA and NRS was poor ($r = 0.47$ and $r = 0.46$, respectively).

Conclusions – The prevalence of malnutrition is high in HIV-positive outpatients. The MNA and NRS questionnaires are not useful in assessing nutritional status in these patients.

The Efficacy of Quick Nutritional Screening

T.M. Semesko, Y.G. Grigorov, S.G. Kozlovskaya and L.L. Sineok

Institute of Gerontology, Kiev, Ukraine

A quick nutritional screen combined with 24-hour recall methodology allows an evaluation of nutrition and health status in a large population. We studied 157 elderly people (60+ years of age) living with their families. The average age of the men was 72 years and of the women, 74 years.

Methods – The 24-hour recall method and a specially devised questionnaire were used to study nutrition and health status. The criterion for risk of inadequate nutrition was an energy intake below accepted norms in Ukraine, that is, <2,100 kcal/day for men and 1,800 kcal/day for women, a dietary protein intake of <0.8 g/kg of body weight, or a combination of these two.

Results – Based on the 24-hour recall method, we found a high risk of inadequate nutrition as reflected in low energy intake: 59% of the men and 56.4% of the women. An insufficient protein intake confirmed the inadequacy of nutrition in 59.6% of the men and 59% of the women.

Conclusions – In evaluating the risk of nutritional deficit, the criterion of energy intake alone was sufficient in the case of males, while we also had to consider protein intake in females.

Nutrition and Health of Elderly Lonely Disabled People Dependent on Social Welfare Services

L.L. Sineok, B.Y. Medovar and L.A. Podust

Institute of Gerontology, Kiev, Ukraine

Socioeconomic changes in Ukraine, which have reduced social guarantees, have affected the quality of life of elderly citizens, especially those living alone. We studied the nutrition of 226 elderly people (60+ years of age) living alone and being served meals in their homes.

Methods – Nutritional status was estimated by the 24-hour recall method plus a questionnaire devised to examine health status, and data from medical examinations.

Results – We found a decrease in consumption of milk products on average by 45%, vegetables by 34%, meat by 60%, and fish by 82% compared with geriatric dietetic norms. As a result, protein intake fell by 35%, fat intake by 48%, and carbohydrate intake by 16%. The dietary provision of vitamins and minerals was reduced. Deficit of vitamin C was 73% and of calcium 71%. In addition, 76% of cases had marked atherosclerotic lesions of the heart and vessels, 73% suffered from ischemic heart disease, 26% had hypertensive disease, and 45% had bone and joint diseases.

Conclusions – Overall, the provision of meals for elderly people in their homes did not meet their nutritional requirements. There is a need to improve the medico-social services for elderly people.

Assessment of the Nutritional State of Elderly Surgical Patients by MNA after Aorto-Coronary Bypass

S. Suzić, V. Starcević, L. Radunović and V. Gal

Institute of Physiology, School of Medicine, Belgrade, Yugoslavia

The prevalence of undernutrition is high in frail elderly people admitted to hospital, as well as in those receiving ambulatory care. Geriatric evaluation should therefore include nutritional assessment. We chose the MNA as a simple, reliable and inexpensive screening tool for nutritional evaluation of ambulatory care patients with hyperlipoproteinemia after aorto-coronary bypass. The patients were studied at least 6 months after their open heart surgery.

Elderly patients (seven women and 18 men) aged over 60 years, with regular control of prothrombin time and plasma lipid levels in our laboratory, were also screened for risk of malnutrition by MNA. Results showed that eight (32%) had scores below 24 (19–23.5), which required additional investigation with biochemical markers such as albumin and cholesterol. In six of the eight cases the risk of malnutrition was confirmed.

Further analyses should be done to evaluate the effects of key factors on the total MNA score from a greater number of patients.

Metabolic and Thermic Responses to Diet and Cold Environment (4 °C) in Obesity during Aging

Orien L. Tulp

Nutrition and Foods, Drexel University, Philadelphia, Pa., USA

To determine the effects of obesity on metabolic and hormonal responses and the capacity for non-shivering thermogenesis during aging, groups of lean and obese LA/Ntul//-*cp* rats were subjected to measures of VO_2 in the young (3–6 months), middle aged (12–16 months), old (24–30 months), and aged (32–36 months; lean only) stages under conditions of thermal neutrality. The VO_2 of lean rats was greater than that of obese, and decreased progressively in both phenotypes at each age studied. In addition, the thermic responses to norepinephrine (100 and 250 µg/kg body weight s.c.), feeding, and acute cold exposure (2–4 °C) also decreased progressively, such that, at the oldest ages, the responses to both diet and environment were no longer present. Food and fluid intakes were consistent with greater lipid utilization with progressive aging, while thyroidal responses were indicative of an age-related T3 resistance in obese animals. Thermic and cold responses to carbohydrate feeding also declined toward zero with progressive aging in both phenotypes.

These results indicate that aging is associated with a progressive decline in the normal dietary and metabolic responses to diet and environment. Moreover, the effects of obesity further exacerbate that decline, and the impact of these physiologic changes of aging and obesity could affect the MNA in aging.

A Nutrition Survey of Elderly People in Estonia

Raivo Vokk and Ede Raagmets

Department of Food Processing, Tallinn Technical University, Estonia

The aim of this study was to estimate nutrient intake in elderly people living in social care homes in Estonia. Daily menus were analyzed using an upgraded computer program (Micro Nutrica – a Finnish database, 1991). The nutrition survey was carried out in three institutions, and 429 persons aged 61–98 years were involved. The consumption of food energy, macro- and micronutrients (including 12 vitamins and 19 minerals) was calculated and compared with Estonian and Scandinavian nutrition recommendations.

An insufficient intake of dietary fiber, vitamins A, C, and D, calcium, and zinc was found. There was overconsumption of saturated fatty acids and sodium.

On the basis of the analysis of the daily menus, recommendations are made for improving nutrient intakes in these elderly people.

Analysis of Hospital Cost and Morbidity in Relation to Nutritional Status of Patients More Than 65 Years Old in a General Surgery Unit

L. Cirafici[a], M. Gillet[a] and P.H. Wiesel[b]

[a]*General Surgery Unit and* [b]*Gastroenterology Division, CHUV, Lausanne, Switzerland*

Many studies have shown a correlation between presurgery nutritional status and post-surgery morbidity. A malnourished patient has more nosocomial problems and stays longer in hospital, with an increase in global hospital cost. European and North American studies show a malnutrition incidence of 30–40% in medical and surgical patients. The Swiss malnutrition incidence is not known.

Patients and Methods – During 1 month, every consecutive patient aged over 65 admitted to the general surgery unit of CHUV in Lausanne was included in the study (37 females and 41 males, average age 76 years). During this period, 261 patients were admitted to the unit. Nutritional evaluation of the patients was conducted using the MNA, with classification into three groups: satisfactory nutritional status; at risk, and malnourished. The two last groups were regrouped by us into a single category: unsatisfactory nutritional status.

Results – The results are shown in the table.

	Nutritional status	
	unsatisfactory	satisfactory
Incidence (n = 78)	28 (36%)	50 (64%)
Emergency admission (n = 39)	20/28 (71%)	19/50 (38%)
Digestive and liver/biliary pathology (n = 49)	22/28 (79%)	27/50 (54%)
Postsurgery complications (n = 18)†	11/28 (39%)	7/50 (14%)
Hospital mortality (n = 3)	2/28 (7%)	1/50 (2%)
5-month follow-up mortality (n = 8)	5/28 (18%)	3/50 (6%)
Hospital average stay, days	18 ± 15	12 ± 7*

* $p < 0.05$.

† Post-surgery complications: parietal abscess, urinary infection, anastamosis leak, transit problem, subdiaphragmatic abcess, infection.

Comment – The incidence of malnutrition in elderly patients in our surgical unit is high, of the same order of magnitude as described in other countries. The majority of patients admitted as emergencies are malnourished. Patients with unsatisfactory nutritional status suffer principally from digestive and liver or biliary tract diseases. These patients will show more nosocomial diseases and will stay longer in hospital. An additional study will be conducted to find out if early nutritional care can decrease morbidity and reduce costs incurred by these malnourished patients.

Nutritional Status in Patients with Leg Ulcers

Ulla Wissing, Mitra Unosson and Anna-Christina Ek

Department of Medicine and Care, Division of Nursing Science, Faculty of Health Sciences, Linkoping University, Linkoping, Sweden

The aim of this study was to assess nutritional status in patients with leg ulcers. The patients were living in their own homes and treatment was given in primary health care. The MNA was used in 50 women and 20 men, mean age 79.7 ± 6.3 years and 77.9 ± 7.0 years, respectively. Thirty-two patients were classified as at risk of malnutrition and two were malnourished. The women had a significantly lower mean total MNA score (22.8 ± 3.0) than the men (24.7 ± 2.4). Patients classified as at risk of malnutrition or malnourished were more often living alone and were more dependent on social home help services compared with the well-nourished. There were no significant differences between the well-nourished patients and those classified as at risk of malnutrition or malnourished with regard to the number and the duration of open ulcers. This study shows that nearly 50% of the patients with leg ulcers were classified as at risk of malnutrition or were malnourished, which may have a negative impact on wound healing.

Conclusion: The MNA Research and Practice

B. Vellas

Department of Internal Medicine and Clinical Gerontology, Toulouse University Hospital, Toulouse, France; Clinical Nutrition Program, University of New Mexico, Albuquerque, N.Mex., USA

When we decided to work on nutrition and aging 10 years ago, we first studied how to assess nutritional status. We found published reports on many kinds of biological, anthropometric, and dietary nutritional indices. If fact, we had problems very similar to those arising with Alzheimer's disease, which is so common in elderly patients – there is no unique marker to assess dementia, but many different measures. However, there is one very valuable aid, a screening tool created by Folstein, the Mini-Mental State examination or the MMS. We decided to use the same kind of approach for nutrition and we designed a tool to assess nutritional status in the elderly: the MNA [1, 2].

The MNA is not a perfect tool for assessing nutritional status in the elderly. It certainly has some deficiencies. However, it is easy to use, cheap, standardized, and can help as a comparative tool as well as a teaching tool for medical students. We should remember that, as with other geriatric assessment tools, it was first created for use with frail elderly people.

We know that malnutrition is very common in elderly people in hospital or living in nursing homes. However, malnutrition is not usually diagnosed in the elderly, and as a result nutritional support is not usually prescribed. To assess frail elderly people we needed a specific and validated tool like the MMS for cognitive function, the geriatric depression scale, the Tinetti gait and balance disorders scale, and the activities of daily living scales (ADL and IADL). Because in the past we did not have tools to assess nutritional status, nutritional evaluation and intervention were not integrated into most of the comprehensive geriatric assessment programs. That is why we decided to create the MNA.

Medicine in the past was purely clinical; physicians had only their hands to examine their patients. Today medicine involves an excessive number of investigations, sometimes dangerous for frail elderly patients and always costly. Intermediate between the medicine of the past and the medicine of today we have the opportunity to introduce a new kind of medicine – modern gerontology, with tools that the primary care physician can use before embarking on more complex investigations. These tools are our new technology. As was shown in the past by Rubenstein [1], geriatric assessment gives us the possibility of reducing morbidity in elderly people and decreasing health care costs (hospital admissions, medical complications, nursing home use), while improving functional capacities and quality of life for frail elderly people. These assessment tools are cheap to use and have resulted in some very important research, as we have seen in this symposium.

Geriatric assessment permits early detection, early intervention, and better results with a decrease in health costs. For example, we know now that, with an MNA score between 17 and 23.5, we can detect elderly persons who are at risk of malnutrition before there is a decrease in weight or plasma albumin. Those with an MNA <17 are more likely to have protein-energy malnutrition with low plasma albumin and weight loss. It will be important for these patients to have oral or enteral nutrition intervention. After every nutritional assessment with the MNA, physicians must *check where patients lose points*. It will then be possible to understand the causes of malnutrition and to propose an appropriate intervention: dietetary supplements, help at home, decrease in drug treatment, and so on.

As we can see from this symposium, we now have much data showing that we can include the MNA as part of the comprehensive geriatric assessment. We need now to increase the numbers of geriatric assessment teams so that there is one in every hospital and to teach the family practitioner and primary care physician how to use the MNA in clinical practice for those of their patients who are frail, who live alone, or who have anorexia or weight loss.

References

1. Vellas B, Guigoz Y, Garry PJ. The Mini Nutritional Assessment. *Facts, research and intervention in geriatrics,* 4th ed. New York: Springer & Serdi Publishing, 1997.
2. Guigoz Y, Vellas B, Garry PJ. Assessing the nutritional status of the elderly: the Mini Nutritional Assessment as part of the geriatric evaluation. *Nutr Rev* 1996; 54: S59–65.

Mini Nutritional Assessment (MNA): Research and Practice in the Elderly:
B. Vellas; P.J. Garry; Y. Guigoz (eds),
Nestlé Nutrition Workshop Series Clinical & Performance Programme, Vol. 1, pp. 177–185,
Nestec Ltd.; Vevey/S. Karger AG, Basel, © 1999.

Discussions of Poster Presentations

Molaschi *et al.* (Dr. Cappa)

Dr. Vellas: Is it a physician or a nurse who does the MNA in the nursing home?

Dr. Cappa: The physician does it.

Dr. Chumlea: You had 24 men. There can be sometime a sex and age interaction, particularly in men. Were the men more severely affected or was there no sex difference in the analysis?

Dr. Cappa: There was no sex difference.

Saletti *et al.* (Ms. Saletti)

Dr. Vellas: I am surprised that 70% of the people living in your nursing homes have an MNA of < 17. In most studies the proportion is < 30%. What is the explanation for this?

Ms. Saletti: People in nursing homes in Sweden tend to be very sick. Maybe that is the explanation. Old people tend to live in service flats, sheltered homes, or old people's homes. The people who live in nursing homes are really in the final stages.

Dr. Rubenstein: So how much of the effect on MNA is due to disease and how much to insufficient nutrition?

Ms. Saletti: I don't know, but from the point of view of a dietician I think there is a lot that we can do with food, and we have developed routines for working with these people.

Dr. Morley: Your proportion of malnourished individuals is very high compared with almost any "free-living" population. This would suggest a problem with nutrition in old people. Why is Sweden, which is supposed to be a good place to live, struggling with its old people? Do you think the food is not well prepared in the nursing homes?

Ms. Saletti: I think they often give the wrong kind of food. They tend to give food that is low in fat and high in fiber.

De Ridder *et al.* (Dr. Vanderbroele)

Dr. Vellas: One problem is that nobody uses the same scores for ADL assessment.

Dr. Vanderbroele: I know. One of the advantages of the MNA is that you have one score which is used by everyone.

Dr. Guesry: You still have a lot of malnourished people who are not identified by the ADL assessment.

Dr. Vanderbroele: Yes, but that's a choice we had to make. We can't carry out MNA on everybody.

Dr. Guesry: This is an important point. Is the test for populations or for individuals? I think this needs further discussion.

Dr. Rubenstein: I was going to make a similar observation. I'm surprised that activities of daily life and malnutrition are so overlapping that one could be a screen for the other, but I think it is an interesting hypothesis. It is an important idea that the MNA may be too long an instrument for general population screening. Maybe we need to do a screening test with follow-up confirmation.

Dr. Vellas: MNA was designed for frail elderly people. If you want a screening test for healthier people, you need other kinds of tools.

Dr. Vanderbroele: Our patients were all sick people receiving home care, so with the chosen cutoff point we actually defined frail people by the ADL assessment.

Dr. Wiesel: In your hands, was MNA suitable for use as a screening test in a large population, or did you find it too difficult to do in patients with recall problems who cannot answer the questions?

Dr. Vanderbroele: I don't think MNA was too difficult. The data were collected by the nurses who were looking after the patients. It motivates them strongly, because it's something new for them, and for the patients too. It gives them something to talk about!

Dr. Morley: Would it not be better to concentrate on people at risk rather than people who are severely malnourished? Particularly in the home care population, there will be a subgroup with severe malnutrition whom you will never be able to help, no matter what you do. It might be better to focus on the people who are on the borderline rather than the ones who are severely malnourished. From a public health point of view, perhaps the worst people are not the best ones to look at.

Dr. Griep: Did you calculate the correlation between the ideal score and risk of malnutrition? Isn't it true that the higher the degree of dependency, the higher the risk of malnutrition?

Dr. Vanderbroele: There is certainly a correlation.

Dr. Henessee: As a nurse, I would like to commend you for this work. I've tried to implement the MNA in home care patients in the USA, but many nurses find it too difficult to do in the home care setting. In the USA it is now a regulatory requirement to screen all home care patients and I'd like to use MNA across the board, but it is a little cumbersome.

Dr. Vanderbroele: I don't want to be too optimistic. This is the first stage of the study. We then have a second stage where we must design the nursing intervention protocol, and then we have to try to make it generally applicable. That part may be the most difficult of all. So we're not there yet.

Dr. Vellas: For healthy elderly people we probably only need a simple, easy-to-apply screening tool, but sick elderly people are so likely to be malnourished and nutritional intervention is so important that the MNA is really necessary. It is a lot of work, but necessary.

Gazzotti *et al.* (Dr. Gazzotti)

Dr. Camilla: Was there any correlation between MNA and the length of the stay in hospital?

Dr. Gazzotti: A very good question, but we don't have these data.

Dr. Vellas: Do you have any data on the reliability of the MNA in your hospital?

Dr. Gazzotti: Yes, we studied interobserver agreement. MNA was done by two clinicians in 40 patients. We measured agreement by the κ coefficient and found that it was significantly different from zero, so we concluded that MNA was a reliable and useful tool in clinical practice.

Dr. Chumlea: Maybe I'm missing something, but in administering the MNA, the observer is passive. The answers are dependent upon the subject, so there should be no observer effect. If all I do is ask you to answer the questions, as an observer I have no effect upon the outcome. The way you ask the questions may add additional variance, but that means that the interpretation of MNA scores from one location to another will then be affected by who is asking the question. That will affect the interpretation of comparisons between two studies. This is an issue that needs looking into.

Dr. Rubenstein: What difficulties did you have in the practical use of MNA?

Dr. Gazzotti: We have had difficulty with patients who can't answer the questions. We have also had problems with three items where there was poor agreement between clinicians, though we don't know why. These were brachial circumference (two clinicians could not agree on this item), hydration score, and the presence of skin ulcers.

Dr. Chumlea: Some physicians and nurses have difficulties in doing the anthropometric measurements. That's normal. The difficulty is that they often don't receive adequate training, and they don't do the measurements often enough to maintain their skills.

Dr. Salvá: What special problems do you have in doing MNA in acute care?

Dr. Gazzotti: The main one is when the patient is confused or disoriented, when it's difficult to get answers.

Dr. Vellas: In such cases you can question the family. That's the way we do it.

Blanchon *et al.* (Dr. Beauchet)

Dr. Guesry: Do you agree that calf circumference is the best variable for this type of assessment?

Dr. Beauchet: Maybe Dr. Chumlea can give us a commentary on calf circumference?

Dr. Chumlea: The amount of data relating calf circumference directly to fat-free mass specifically in the elderly is not that large. The data at present mainly involve relations reported in surveys that were not actually measuring body composition. In those studies, individuals who had been active had a decrease in calf circumference, though not of arm circumference, as their activity level decreased. Our own studies of changes in fat-free mass, and several other smaller studies, appear to support this, but there are no large studies at present. The available reference data for calf circumference are primarily from the studies we've done in the United States and from the studies in Toulouse, France, and those that have been reported here. There are some calf circumference data from the health examination surveys conducted by the National Center for Health Statistics in the early 1960s, and calf circumferences will be included in NHANES IV, which will start next year.

Dr. Cohendy: In postoperative patients I would definitely not use serum albumin as a nutritional indicator, particularly after fractured neck of femur, because of the quantities of fluid that are likely to be given to patients during and after the operation. Secondly in postoperative patients, I would be quite reluctant to use calf circumference because of the high incidence of leg vein thrombosis. In such cases variation in the diameter of the calf is directly related to the deep vein thrombosis and has nothing to do with nutritional state. These kinds of results, in my opinion, should be treated with caution.

Dr. Guesry: You don't systematically give prophylaxis against deep venous thrombosis?

Dr. Cohendy: Recent studies have shown that in this kind of surgery, even with prophylaxis, for example low molecular weight heparin and early mobilization, the amount of the deep vein thrombosis remains very high, more than 20%.

Dr. Camilla: I am still puzzled by your comment that you consider calf circumference to be a good indicator of chronic undernutrition because elderly people have many reasons for edema and hence an increased calf circumference.

Dr. Beauchet: I agree, but in our small study we excluded all patients with any pathology that could cause calf edema, such as phlebitis, renal insufficiency and cardiac failure. However, we found it difficult to assess the role of immobilization on calf muscle volume. Although I have no proof of the reliability of my data, I have three indirect arguments to back me up: (1) the immobilization period in our patients was very short, on average 8 days; (2) we measured the opposite calf to the femoral neck fracture; (3) we instituted a very early program of exercise, with twice daily isometric contractions to limit the decrease in muscle volume during immobilization

It must be admitted as well that our control group was at the lower limit of the distribution of the anthropometric norms published by Vellas *et al.* in 1992 [1]. This could explain the albumin value. I believe it also gives added confidence to our calf circumference and MNA results. Moreover, when we measure calf circumference we assess muscle mass and lean body mass, which is directly related to wasting and decreased muscle strength following falls and fractures.

Because of the indirect nature of our arguments we will be conducting a second study involving the patients very early, before surgery.

Khavinson and Solovieva (Dr. Khavinson)

Dr. Guigoz: Do you have measures of albumin in your patients?

Dr. Khavinson: No, we measured that in a previous study. This study was specifically to investigate immunological indices in this kind of patient.

Dr. Vellas: You found some significant differences between the MNA results and immunological function that we did not find in Toulouse. Do you have the mean MNA scores in the three groups? What was the mean MNA in people with a score of <17?

Dr. Khavinson: It was 12. And in people whose MNA was >23, it was 28.

Dr. Vellas: That may be the explanation. In the nursing home patients in Toulouse the mean MNA was nearer 25, certainly not as high as 28.

Dr. Guesry: In your conclusion, you propose the use of T lymphocyte function as an additional variable in MNA. Do you really think that it is practical? How much does it cost and how long does it take? How easy is it to obtain this type of measurement? After all, MNA was designed to be done easily by a non-specialized person at the bedside. It has to be cheap and fast.

Dr. Khavinson: Our hope was that this could improve the precision of MNA.

Dr. Morley: I'm happy to see that the CD4/CD8 ratio reflected the MNA score, because that is the one thing that is specific for malnutrition as people get older. The way we have used the CD4/CD8 ratio in St. Louis is in people who look very malnourished, if we are having trouble treating them. People with a low CD4/CD8 ratio often need 10 or 20 days of antibiotics before they get better, and they have more atypical infections. So I would see this measurement as a treatment indicator, as in AIDS patients. I would not go straight to T cell measurement.

Dr. Rea: I'd like to confirm what Dr. Morley has been saying. In a large study in Northern Ireland of 80- and 90-year-olds, we found a 10% incidence of CD4 lymphopenia in healthy elderly people living in the community. And although we did not have information then about MNA status, we do know that the CD4 count correlated with BMI, weight, and cholesterol. I suppose those measures are similar to the measures of malnutrition that are being measured in the MNA.

Dr. Khavinson: I would like to make one comment. It is well known that thymic function declines with age. From our immunological investigations, it was also clear that the T lymphocyte function and T cell numbers decrease with age, and we noted that the state of malnutrition was correlated with lymphocyte function and the function of the thymus. We carried out an *in vitro* study in which we treated lymphocyte cultures with thymus extract and showed an improvement in the function of T lymphocytes. Maybe the way to help these malnourished people is to use a food additive derived from thymus extract in order to normalize their T cell function.

Maaravi *et al.* (Dr. Maaravi)

Dr. Vellas: I think it is really important that a nutritional assessment is part of a comprehensive geriatric assessment. This is straightforward for geriatricians, because they are used to doing geriatric assessments, and it's easy to add one tool. It's more difficult for nutritionists, because they have no experience in geriatric assessment.

Dr. Guesry: You said you modified the MNA. Could you tell us how you modified it, and to what extent? I was interested to see that your correlation with mortality was poor, or rather nonexistent, with $p = 0.7$. Dr. Guigoz got a much better correlation. I wonder whether in your modification you have lost something important. At the start of this meeting I said that it would be nice to have one tool that is used by everybody, so that we can compare studies. However, I think we have had more communications on modified MNA than we have on MNA. I'm worried that these many changes may make comparisons difficult.

Dr. Maaravi: As I explained, at the time we designed our study, we did not know about the MNA. We extracted from our data as many items as possible that are collected in the MNA and the modification was not great: we are only missing some of the data from the dietary block. As to mortality, we are considering relatively healthy free-living 70-year-olds whom we have been following for two years. This is too short a time for reliable mortality statistics. We are conducting a second stage of this longitudinal study on a larger scale. We are going to use the complete original MNA, and I hope we will have more results to present the next time we meet.

Dr. Guesry: My comment did not reflect a desire to sell the MNA, only to have a common language!

Dr. Morley: You should not apologize for the modified MNA; we will present our one tomorrow! Our data are very similar to yours, and the important message is that a good nutritional assessment tool can predict frailty and health care utilization, which is something we can intervene in. Thus it is very important to pick out the nutritional component. We can argue whether or not the MNA, or other tools, truly picks out nutrition or whether it identifies something else, but clearly a large component *is* nutrition, and we are showing that nutrition is an extremely important factor in poor outcomes for older people.

Dr. Maaravi: We are planning to put MNA into routine practice in our services, that is, the geriatric emergency department, the geriatric rehabilitation department, and home care services.

Dr. Vanderbroele: You specifically mentioned the correlation between MNA and cardiac disease. Was this one of your modifications and did you screen other systems or diseases?

Dr. Maaravi: Our study was on a very large scale. We had thousands of variables from all chronic diseases that we thought could be correlated with nutritional status. The ones that I presented were the ones that yielded correlations. Having ischemic heart disease can influence your nutritional state or *vice versa.* We studied many other diseases and could not find other correlations.

McDowell *et al.* (Dr. Rea)

Dr. Vellas: When we use MNA in clinical practice, we have to be careful about the scores. For example, someone with a score of 23 is not necessarily at risk of malnutrition. It is the same as with Mini Mental State. People scoring 26.5 or 26 on Mini Mental State do not necessarily have dementia. We need to be careful about that.

Dr. Rea: I'm saying that this group is at risk.

Dr. Vellas: I don't know if people with a score of 23 are really at risk. Maybe.

Dr. Arnaud-Battandier: What did you do with your patients who were malnourished?

Dr. Rea: Nothing to date, because they are living in the community. The MNA is just a tool. I've also looked at BMI in 90-year-olds in the community and found that 10% of them have a BMI of <18.5. So many of these elderly people are apparently well, it's very hard to know what to do. Will we harm them by introducing nutritional supplements, or by causing worries about their health? If they have already survived to 90, maybe we should not interfere.

Dr. Rubenstein: You seem to be making a fairly large distinction over relatively small differences in means. A small proportion of people with very low scores will of course bring your mean down. I was also struck by the relatively high percentage of people "at risk" compared with some of the other studies presented today. You said that there were many people who had only one or two meals a day, but I wasn't sure whether this was a cultural difference. Maybe people in your area always eat two meals a day, and therefore automatically lose a point on the scale. Is this merely a cultural difference or do you think they are really at risk?

Dr. Rea: I'm not sure whether they are at risk, given that so many of them are apparently well and living in the community. Perhaps the MNA is not a sensitive enough indicator for people at risk. In other words, it may be picking up too many people. I began to use the tool simply because we had found that 10% of 90-year-olds had CD4 lymphopenia, which does seem to be associated with undernutrition. I wanted a simple screening tool to see if I could pick out these people. I have not gone on to put those two groups together, but there does seem to be a rather large number of people in this "at risk" group, which I was a bit concerned about.

Dr. Guesry: Is MNA too sensitive?

Dr. Guigoz: I don't think it is too sensitive. I have the impression that the "at risk" people form an unstable population. So some will stay as they are, others will go up to the normal range, but most will probably have an event which will cause them to decline into the malnourished range. It would be interesting to follow up your subjects who were at risk during this study.

Dr. Charles: In the Irish Republic, as opposed to Northern Ireland, there is a great scarcity of information on nutritional status of the elderly. We are at present trying to get together a food and nutrition policy for the elderly on a national level. I'd like to comment about the eating habits of Irish people, which could have a lot to do with nutritional intakes. Traditionally we are a population that has relied in the past on a certain limited number of foods. I would prefer the MNA to be too sensitive for the Irish population, because at the moment we have a huge problem in identifying malnutrition among the elderly. If it is too sensitive, for me that's good because that means I get referrals rather that not getting them! I'd like to ask whether you think that the MNA is a good measure of nutritional status for the Irish?

Dr. Rea: I'm not sure.

Dr. Chumlea: You showed a sex difference. How many of the men were widowers and how many still had a living spouse? Normally, the men who live longest tend to have their wives with them still.

Dr. Rea: I can't say for MNA, but when we looked at BMI in elderly men, there did seem to be a difference. BMI in elderly men who lived alone was lower than it was in those who lived with someone else, regardless of who that was. As you would know, there are not as many 90-year-old men living in the community as women, so we had a limited group to do statistics on.

Dr. Salvá: I did not understand how you selected the population?

Dr. Rea: The population of the greater Belfast area is 250,000 people. We wrote to all the general practitioners and asked them if they would allow us access to their patients who were over 90 (that was initially, because the 90-year-olds were done first): in that group we were given perhaps 200 or 300 names. We then approached the practices who helped us the first time, and asked for access to the 80-year-olds, and we selected these randomly. The study is ongoing; this is only a small part of what is happening.

Dr. Morley: There have been other studies from Ireland which have shown nutrient deficiency. Ireland looks worse than many other places, and there are two factors that I wonder about: one is the use of alcohol which may be high; the other is depression. Certainly when you look at Belfast, there are reasonable grounds for a high incidence of depression. Have you looked at those two as potential causes?

Dr. Rea: I have information on alcohol intake. There is no difference in alcohol intake between 70-, 80- and 90-year-olds. I don't have information comparing them with the rest of the population. I don't know about the geriatric depression scale. All I know is that all these people could score at least 28 and higher on what is the equivalent of the Fallstein mini mental score. So they were mentally competent, and they were going to get 1 on the MNA for that.

Piquet *et al.* (Dr. Piquet)

Dr. Schwenk: I have two questions. First, you chose the absolute value of body cell mass as a reference. What was you rationale for that? Body weight is generally used as the reference? Second, did you look to see whether individual questions within the MNA had better predictive value than total MNA? Nobody among us will be very surprised that the MNA did not perform very well in this particular population, since it was developed for the geriatric population.

Dr. Piquet: In answer to the first question, we took dry lean body mass as the reference norm. These values come from Geneva and were derived from a large scale study on several thousand people. They are not yet published but I hope they will be soon. As to your second question, various factors such as not living independently, or needing help to perform social activities were strongly correlated with end-stage chronic disease, not surprisingly, but generally the correlation was poor.

Dr. Vellas: We have tried to use bioelectrical impedance as a reference value, but we had strange results in sick malnourished patients. Do you think bioelectrical impedance is a useful measurement in sick patients with malnutrition?

Dr. Piquet: The problem with malnutrition is that the patient may be overhydrated. We use BIA only if there is no problem with hydration. In old patients we also have the problem of norms for BIA.

Dr. Vellas: Because there are very few studies of BIA in patients with malnutrition.

Dr. Ferry: What kind of bioelectrical impedance did you use? There is a difference between one frequency, two frequency, or multi-frequency.

Dr. Piquet: We used one frequency.

Dr. Ferry: So Dr. Vellas was right when he said it was difficult to obtain a good impedance value with one frequency. I think Dr. Chumlea will agree with me.

Dr. Chumlea: The issue is between single frequency impedance measurement and the newer multifrequency impedance measurement that technically allows you to separate intracellular and extracellular fluids. Much work has been done with the single frequency and the work with the multifrequency impedance is just starting to be published. The question that Dr. Vellas was addressing was the use of impedance in elderly populations or in clinical populations. The problem has been that most of the work has been done in healthy normal populations, and has then been applied to clinical populations. That's always the wrong way to do it. Kotler *et al.* [2] have done a lot of very good work with impedance in patients with HIV and have developed certain specific equations, validating the technique in these patients. So that's the way to do it. The other issue is that prediction equations have a standard error of the estimate for a group and a standard error of the estimate for an individual, which is not always quoted. Once you start using the equations on individuals, the standard error can become greatly inflated. Thus a prediction of 20% body fat may have a standard error in the individual of ± 10%, so the variance around that prediction can be very large. You need to be very careful in using it.

Dr. Rubenstein: Did you do some individual question analysis to find out why the MNA was not working in AIDS patients? Was it perhaps because of malabsorption, so the patients were eating enough but nothing was absorbed, thus making the food intake question unhelpful, or was there some other factor involved?

Dr. Piquet: I think that malabsorption may have played a role, because most of our patients have diarrhea.

Dr. Cohendy: I believe that subjective evaluation will have decreased the MNA score in these patients. They were all taking at least three to five drugs, and all of them knew that they were very sick. If you ask them: Do you believe that your health is better than that of your neighbor?, they will obviously answer no. So many of them will lose points in the MNA evaluation. In my opinion this decreases the power of the MNA in this kind of patient.

Dr. Morley: Beside the bioelectrical impedance problem, people with AIDS have low testosterones, and because of that they develop loss of muscle mass. So you cannot rely on anthropometric measurement – even midarm circumference may be a poor measurement of malnutrition in this particular population. I would have concluded from your study that MNA may be better than the classical measurements for this population.

Dr. Vellas: It is good that this study was done in adults. In the past, geriatric medicine has taken a lot from other specialties; now it is other specialties that have taken something from geriatrics.

Ciraffici *et al.* (Dr. Wiesel)

Dr. Cohendy: What was the nutritional management of these postoperative patients, in particular the emergency patients?

Dr. Wiesel: The nutritional care of the patients was very poor. Most of the patients had no nutritional support, some had TPN. In this surgical department there were plans to change nutritional support from TPN to enteral feeding or oral feeding, but that had not taken place when the study was done in 1995. Things have changed now, and there is less TPN and more enteral feeding. We plan to do a study in which one group of patients is managed by a nutritional team and another by the surgeons.

Dr. Miller: It seems to me that you have a very nice setup to take the important next step, which is to start to tease apart the MNA and rebuild it to some extent according to what it shows about the type of patients who can respond to nutritional intervention and do well.

Dr. Camilla: Since there is no gold standard for nutritional assessment and MNA might be better for this group, did you compare it with subjective global assessment?

Dr. Wiesel: I did not show the data, because we could not do this in all the patients. We tried, but we only achieved it in two thirds of the group and the correlation was poor. The subjective assessments were poorly done, mainly because of lack of training which introduced bias. The purpose of our study was to get nurses to do a nutritional assessment using the easy parts of the MNA. We think it could be an easy tool without the biological measurements – that is, using only the questionnaire components and measuring the easy things.

References

1. Vellas B, Chumlea WC, Béziat F, Ghisolfi-Marque A, Guo S, Conceicao J, Sédeuilh M, Dufetelle R, Albarède JL. Etude des normes anthropométriques dans une population française de 492 personnes âgées en bonne santé et vivant à domicile. L'Année Gérontologique. Paris: Serdi Publishing Co, 1992: 203–217.
2. Kotler DP, Burastero S, Wang J, Pierson RN Jr. Prediction of body cell mass, fat-free mass, and total body water with bioelectrical impedance analysis: effects of race, sex, and disease. *Am J Clin Nutr* 1996; 64 (suppl): 489S–97S.

Mini Nutritional Assessment (MNA): Research and Practice in the Elderly:
B. Vellas; P.J. Garry; Y. Guigoz (eds),
Nestlé Nutrition Workshop Series Clinical & Performance Programme, Vol. 1, pp. 187–190,
Nestec Ltd.; Vevey/S. Karger AG, Basel, © 1999.

Conclusion

When we started working on nutrition and aging in Toulouse, we worked first on nutritional markers. Our problem was that there were too many nutritional markers: anthropometry; biological markers, bioelectric impedance, DEXA, and so on. We had the same kind of problem with dementia and Alzheimer disease. There is no unique marker for Alzheimer disease, so we needed a reliable means of neuropsychological assessment. A very useful tool turned out to be the Mini Mental State Examination (MMSE). We felt that if we could design a tool like the MMSE for nutrition, this might be a helpful part of geriatric assessment, since at the time nutritional assessment did not feature in most geriatric assessments. We met Yves Guigoz at the World Congress of Gerontology Association in Acapulco 8 years ago, and we corresponded with him about this aim. As a result he visited us in Toulouse and we started collaborative work on the MNA.

The MNA has the same problems as the MMSE – it is not a perfect tool. We had no ambition to design a perfect tool, but we wanted a tool that could be helpful. When the MMSE was first presented to neurologists, most of them said that they did not need it. They claimed they could make a clinical diagnosis of Alzheimer disease without the MMSE. But for most general practitioners without detailed knowledge of Alzheimer disease, the tool was very useful.

The MNA follows the same kind of plan. We wanted a tool that was easy to perform, cheap, standardized (for use in comparing data), and useful in teaching. The teaching role is very important, because residents and fellows as well as dieticians need to learn how to do anthropometric measurements, how to assess body mass index, and how to provide nutritional intervention. We know now that in some big hospitals in the USA malnutrition was recognized in <40% of patients, while nutritional support was given to few of them, though a diagnosis of malnutrition on discharge was never mentioned. That is why there is a lot of work to be done in this area, and physicians, residents and fellows all need additional training. To encourage this, you need a tool. We have tools for cognitive function, we have tools for affective function, we have tools for autonomy; we now needed a tool for nutrition.

What I would like you to remember is that in the past medicine was purely clinical: the physician had only his hands to cure the patient. Now, medicine is too paraclinical: we have too many investigations. What does a physician do when he sees a patient? He orders clinical chemistry, he orders radiology, he orders hematology. The problem is that the social security systems are reluctant to pay for these tests. Geriatric assessment paves the way towards a new type of medicine, one that lies between the purely clinical and the overinvestigative. This geriatric assessment is our new technology for geriatric medicine. We know now from the work of Larry Rubenstein that geriatric assessment can reduce morbidity and be cost-effective. We need to show that this type of geriatric assessment represents a truly new technology by adequate validatory research, as presented in this meeting.

This tool is also cheap. This is the right direction to be moving in, both for medicine and for social security systems. We believe that geriatric assessments need to be the same in different countries. If you go to Toulouse, to New York, or to Mexico City and have your blood pressure taken, everybody does it the same way. We need comparable standardization for geriatric assessment so that we can collect comparative data. Geriatric assessment is a means of early detection, early intervention, and improved results. In elderly people, if we intervene too late, this generates additional problems. This is very important.

When we work on geriatric assessment, we need to think about intervention. If the MNA score is around 24 points, we need to suggest ideas on improving the quality and quantity of the food intake. If the MNA is <17, it generally means there is protein-energy malnutrition. Such people will have low albumin and weight loss, and we must increase the patient's weight and follow other biological markers. For people with a score between 17 and 22.5, there is the possibility of detecting malnutrition before the onset of weight loss, and before there is low albumin. Under such circumstances intervention will be more successful. We also need to look carefully at the areas where patients lose points: for example, if they suffer from weight loss, we need to look at the cause of the weight loss; if they take more than three drugs, we have to look at what kind of drugs are being given and whether they can be changed or discontinued; if there is a mobility disorder, we need to determine what help can be provided; or if there is depression, this can be treated.

In relation to dietetic assessment, if we find patients who are having only one or two meals a day, we need to help them. If we find people who eat little in the way of fruit or vegetables, we must encourage them to take more, since there are many data showing how important it is to eat these foods. Such interventions are a really important part of the MNA.

To finish, I would say that geriatric assessment takes time, but good medicine takes time also, and we must not forget that this is our technology. A gastroenterologist who wants to do a gastroscopy will have to take time to do it, but the gastroscopy will be very useful.

In the future we may need to have two assessments: a short form for healthy elderly people and a longer form for frail people. But the question remains as to whether or not we need to screen healthy elderly people. We know that the prevalence of malnutrition will be very low in such people, only 2–5%, and it may be best to reserve MNA for those people who experience weight loss or anorexia. We need to do more work on the value of the short form of assessment for healthy elderly people.

For frail elderly people, we need two things. The first is a geriatric team, because we cannot expect everybody to do geriatric assessment. Not everybody can do a gastroscopy; there is no one who can do everything. Maybe the best way would be to build up the expertise on geriatric assessment in hospitals. Secondly, for the family practitioner or private practitioner, we need to negotiate with our social security system over how it might be possible to pay for or to reimburse this kind of geriatric assessment. We can work towards convincing the social services that it is better to fund this kind of assessment than to fund excessive numbers of expensive and often unnecessary chemical and radiological tests.

Finally, I would like to thank Nestlé Clinical Nutrition for their support in developing MNA from the start.

B. Vellas

Subject Index